Dear Mary Rose

Now you can look at gardens in a different light.

I hope you enjoy it.

Love

Rob
x

13th May 1993

THE
HEALING
GARDEN

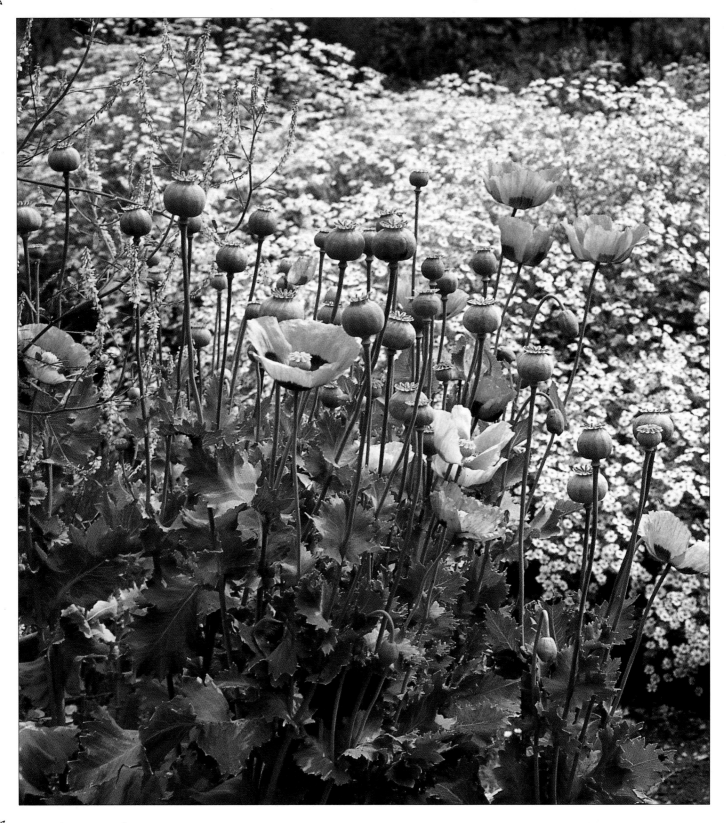

THE HEALING GARDEN

A natural haven for emotional and physical well-being

❧ **SUE MINTER** ❧

Curator of the Chelsea Physic Garden

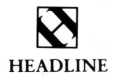

HEADLINE

To Penny with thanks and to all the staff and volunteers
of the Chelsea Physic Garden.

PUBLISHER'S NOTE

Many of the plants mentioned in this book are of medicinal use. However, their
description as such is no indication of their safety and we strongly recommend
consultation with a qualified medical practitioner before using them.

First published in 1993
by HEADLINE BOOK PUBLISHING PLC

10 9 8 7 6 5 4 3 2 1

British Library Cataloguing in Publication Data
Minter, Sue
  Healing Garden: Natural Haven for Emotional and Physical Well-being
  I. Title
  635

ISBN 0-7472-0656-2

AN EDDISON • SADD EDITION
Original concept by Geraldine Christy
Edited, designed and produced by
Eddison Sadd Editions Limited
St Chad's Court
146B King's Cross Road
London WC1X 9DH

Phototypeset in Diotima and Optima by
Dorchester Typesetting, Dorset, England
Origination by Columbia Offset, Singapore
Produced by Mandarin Offset, printed and bound in Hong Kong

HEADLINE BOOK PUBLISHING PLC
Headline House
79 Great Titchfield Street
London W1P 7FN

PHOTOGRAPH ON PAGE 2   *Three important drug plants: the opium poppy, which yields morphine;*
yellow melilot, whose action was copied in the development of antithrombotic drugs; and feverfew,
which is used for migraine.

CONTENTS

o

Preface 7

CHAPTER ONE

THE HEALING ARTS

A marriage of botany and medicine 9

The Ancient Art of Healing 10
Balancing the Humours 12
Folk Medicine 14
The Physic Garden Tradition 16
The Apothecaries' Garden of Simples 18
Medicinal Herbs and Herbalism 20
Homoeopathic Natural Cures 22
Saving the World's Flora 24
Stress: A Hidden Killer? 27
Gaia: A New World View 28

CHAPTER TWO

THE BODY PHYSICAL

Nature's pharmacy 31

Healthy Eating 34
Organic Gardening 37
Growing Healthy Vegetables 40
Fresh Fruit 42
A Wider Range of Fruit and Vegetables 44
Garlic: The Heal-All 48
Medicinal Herbs 50
Herbal Teas to Refresh and Heal 52
Designing a Herb Garden 54
Growing Medicinal Plants for Ornament 58
The Bach Flower Remedies 66

CHAPTER THREE

THE SENSES AWAKENED

Experience enhanced 69

The Mainstay Culinary Herbs 72
Some Delicious Recipes With Herbs 76
Drying and Storing Herbs 78
Mustard: A Condiment and a Medicine 80
Designing With Colour 82

Colour and Mood 84
A Harmony of Warm Colours 86
Complementary Blues and Yellows 88
Structure and Shape 92
The Special Effect of a White Garden 94
Healing Sounds in the Garden 96
The Sound of Running Water 99
What is Scent? 102
Planning Scent in Your Garden 106
Lavender 109
Essential Oils and Aromatherapy 110
The Strewing of Herbs and
Scenting of the Air 112
The Texture of Plants 114
A Garden for the Partially Sighted 116
Plant Treatments to Make You Feel Good 118

CHAPTER FOUR

A SPIRITUAL HAVEN

The search for paradise 121

The Secret Garden 124
Garden Design: Nature and Order 127
A Formal Garden 128
The Art of Topiary 130
A Romantic Garden 132
Still Water: Pools for Contemplation 134
The Mystical Maze 138
Sculpture in the Garden 140
The Urban Wildlife Garden 144
A Place for Self-Expression 147
A Japanese Garden 148
A Town Mediterranean Garden 150
The Therapy of Gardening 153
The End of the Day 154

Further Reading 156
Addresses and Suppliers 157
Index 158
Acknowledgements 160

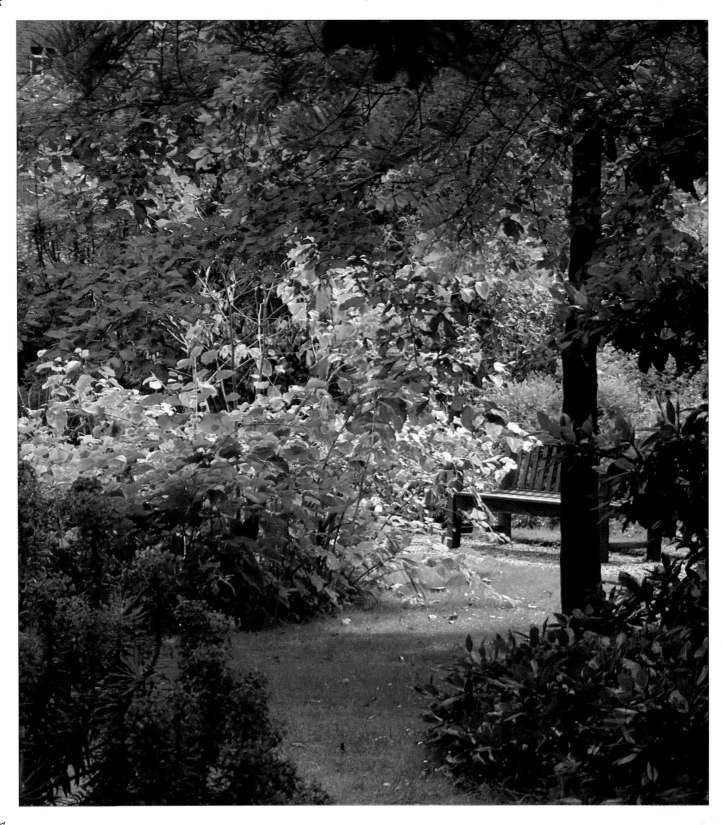

PREFACE

'All life on earth depends on plants', yet many of us only realize this simple truth through contact with plants in our gardens. And, for many, the healing properties of plants are hidden behind the way modern medicine presents them in pill form.

This book attempts to put plants back at the forefront of medicine and also to broaden the definition of healing to include the way that the garden is used for recreation, self-expression and creative interplay with the natural world.

For people working with the soil throughout the world our dependence on plants is a fact of everyday life – almost 'is' life itself – and so it is common to find rural societies with a highly developed sense of how to care for the environment and conserve it, in the belief that the land is 'not ours but borrowed from our children to come'. This seamless thread of awareness is lost in more 'modern' urban societies and causes a need to reconnect, to 'get away from the concrete' in a park, a green open space, a garden.

This is a broad book, an attempt to make connections between ideas about healing and how they link with plants. It does not attempt to promote or endorse any system of healing, rather to review the many ideas that humanity has produced about what illness is and how plants have been enlisted to help. It is also a practical book for the gardener, much of it based on my own experience, and attempts to give a taste of how to create garden features, plan plantings and use plants to create a garden which is healing for you as an individual.

Throughout the book recurs the theme of the five senses of sight, hearing, touch, taste and smell. This is because it is our senses which reconnect us with the natural world and through which we can experience the garden as a healing place. The book also considers the spiritual side of garden-making, with glimpses of how certain traditions of garden design have expressed the psychological needs of the societies which produced them and how we can borrow from these in our own gardens for personal self-expression.

As I write I am aware both of how the many volunteers at the Chelsea Physic Garden gain personal benefit from their connection with these acres, and of how many pharmaceutical companies are beating a path to the Garden's doors with a renewed fervour to take a fresh look at the healing properties of plants. Perhaps this is a renewed recognition of the value of the world of plants and what it can offer us, which augers well for an age which is struggling to contain the many pressures on our environment. Let us hope so.

Sue Minter
October 1992

A corner of the Chelsea Physic Garden
in London, a place to relax
amid urban stress.

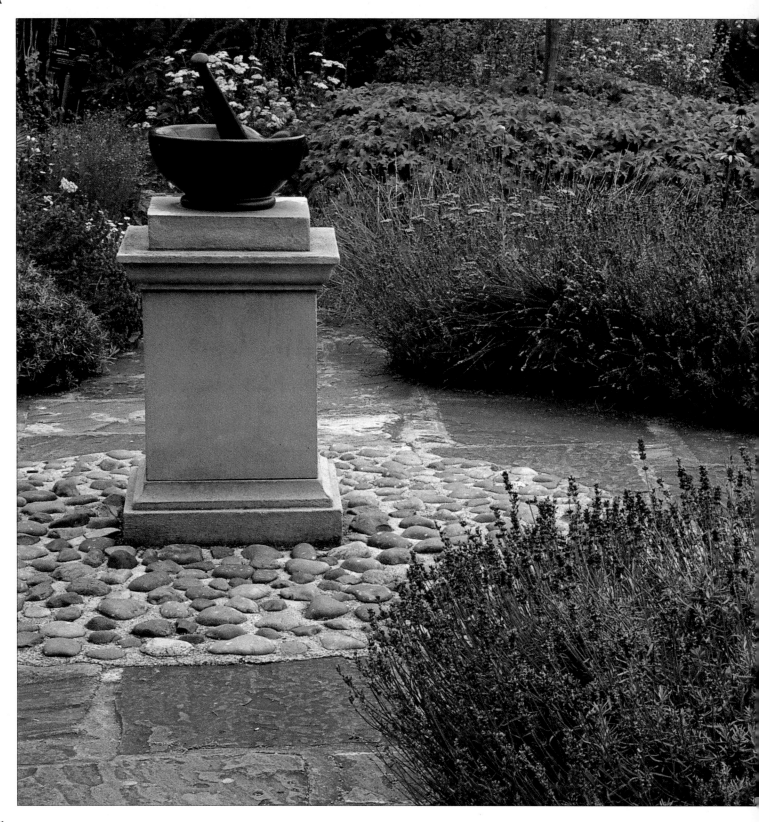

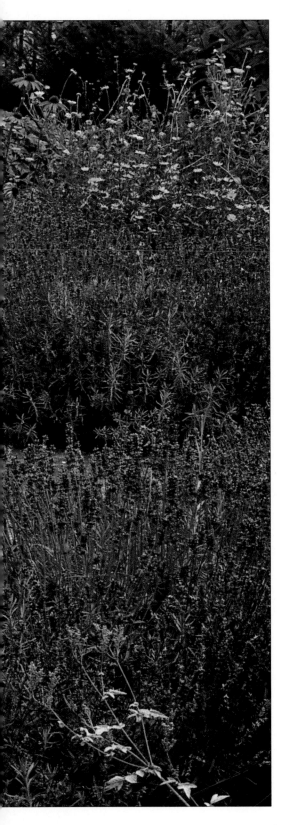

CHAPTER ONE

THE HEALING ARTS

○

A marriage of botany and medicine

'There is no illness but there is a plant to cure it.' This belief was at the root of all medicine from ancient Alexandria through to Renaissance Europe. The entire countryside was nature's pharmacy, and healers identified their plants by descriptions and illustrations in medicinal handbooks known as herbals.

Monastery, guild and university 'physic' gardens were established so that 'physicians' could study and use the principal healing plants collected together in one place. From these gardens developed the modern botanic garden.

Today many societies all over the world still understand the importance of plants in medicine and either grow them for their own use, collect them from the wild or trade in them in medicinal plant markets. As the consumer of a capsule, tablet or ampoule you are less likely to be aware of how these medicines have been derived from plants. The likelihood is that the majority are 'green medicines'.

The apothecary's pestle and mortar sundial in this modern physic garden is a reminder of the traditional role of such gardens in the study of the healing properties of the plants grown there.

THE ANCIENT ART OF HEALING

Over the centuries answers to the question 'What is healing?' have ranged from the purely practical to complex philosophies based on the relation of human beings to the natural, religious or supernatural 'world order'. Cultures have differed in their systems of healing although many have stressed the maintenance of some sort of balance within the individual, a concept not lost on today's New Age 'seekers after health'. Almost without exception, however, all cultures have used plants in some way to cure ailments and prevent illness.

The beginnings of medicine

For the cultures that developed from the Middle Eastern cradles of civilization the earliest roots of medicine lay in Mesopotamia, from 4000 to 1500 BC, where disease was thought to be inflicted by the gods and treatment was by exorcism. From 2000 BC, however, this supernatural approach was gradually superseded by an attention to symptoms that were treated both by propitiating charms and by plant-based medicines.

The Egyptians also maintained parallel beliefs in the supernatural and in the natural causes of illness, and developed the widespread cultivation of drug plants, becoming the chief exporters of opium in Roman times. They were the first to use senna and castor oil as laxatives, and physicians such as Imhotep of the Third Dynasty were famous for prescribing drugs in association with religious rituals. Their patron was Thoth, the scribe god of knowledge, and they established a renowned medical library in the city of Alexandria.

Greek and Roman healing

In Greece, Aristotle (384–322 BC) played down the importance of the supernatural and developed a 'logical' view of the human body being composed of four 'humours', an idea that was first proposed by the many authors of the *Hippocratic Corpus* of the fifth century BC. These liquids (blood, phlegm, yellow bile and black bile) were in balance and affected the body as a microcosm of the world order just as earth, air, fire and water affected the world itself, the macrocosm. It is easy to see how these concepts later became translated into medieval and Renaissance views on alchemy and astrology. Paralleling Aristotle's philosophical ideas

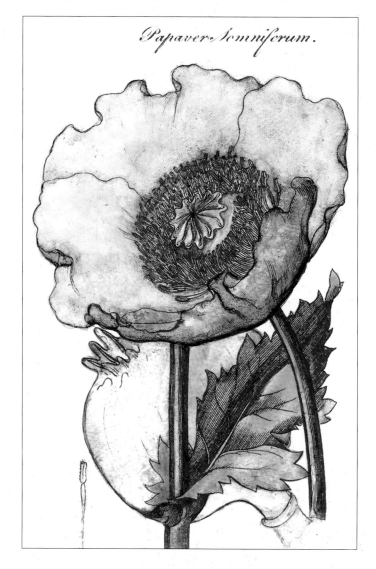

Papaver Somniferum.

The opium poppy yields the painkiller morphine. Its latex has been used as an analgesic since centuries BC.

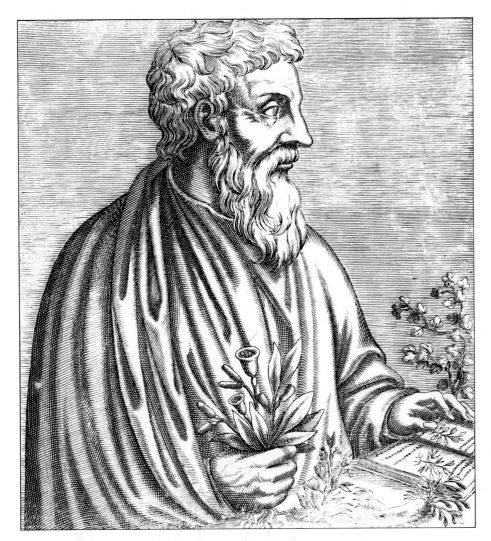

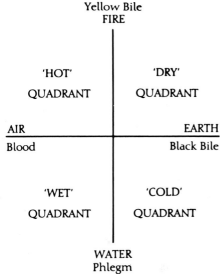

Yellow Bile
FIRE

| 'HOT' | 'DRY' |
| QUADRANT | QUADRANT |

AIR   EARTH
Blood   Black Bile

| 'WET' | 'COLD' |
| QUADRANT | QUADRANT |

WATER
Phlegm

on the maintenance of health through balancing the humours, was the work of Theophrastus (371–287 BC), who described over 550 species of plants and their medicinal uses in maintaining this balance. The Greeks also dedicated temples to the healer god Asclepius as centres of healing, and at the sanctuary of Epidaurus votive offerings modelled on the part of the body cured would be displayed.

The Romans based their medical systems on those of the Greeks. Their most notable source was *De Materia Medica*, by Dioscorides (AD 40–90), the army doctor from Asia Minor, in which he discussed the medicinal use of over 600 plants, including belladonna, calamine and opium.

Dioscorides illustrated from nature the plants he used and his book became standard in Europe well into medieval times. It was used by the Greek physician Galen (AD 129–199), who refined Aristotle's ideas for his practice in Rome and developed a coherent system of physiology and anatomy.

The traditions of the Greeks and Romans survived the Dark Ages following the fall of Rome largely through their use in the Islamic world. In Persia, the physician Avicenna (AD 980–1087) preserved the work of Galen and Aristotle and advanced drug therapy considerably with his complex blending of ingredients, most of which remained plant based.

BALANCING THE HUMOURS

After the fall of Rome the main medical theories continued to follow the principle of the Aristotelian humours and the work of Dioscorides provided a source of reference for plant-based drugs. The treatment of illnesses consisted of restoring the 'balance of the humours' by purging, by various forms of blood-letting (bleeding and cupping) and by the medicinal use of herbs. Diagnosis was made by studying the patient's urine. In the Christian tradition offerings were often made to saints to invoke their protection against disease, while fragrant oils from plants were used to fumigate rooms to ward off the plague (see page 112).

Renaissance learning and discovery

During the Renaissance (1300–1600) enormous conceptual changes radically affected medical thought. On the one hand the idea of the body as a machine was developing, clearly illustrated in the drawings of Leonardo da Vinci (1452–1519) and later in the writings of the French philosopher and mathematician René Descartes (1596–1650). This stimulated medical knowledge by encouraging dissection (the first anatomy theatre was opened in Padua in 1594) which in turn led to a development in medical instruments.

On the other hand there was a growing interest in astrology based on the Hippocratic and Aristotelian views of the human being as a microcosm that is affected by the analogous macrocosm of the heavens. Alchemy was also rooted in the microcosm and macrocosm theory. The Swiss physician Paracelsus (1493–1541) believed that the body functioned as a model of the chemical reactions of the entire universe. Since illnesses were due to chemical imbalance, they could be cured by treating the patient with chemicals. These included mercury and antimony, now known to be highly toxic. The most widely known medical astrologer, famed for his book *The English Physician* (1653), was the herbalist Nicholas Culpeper, who extensively promoted the use of plants for medicinal use.

The real development in plant-based medicine, however, came not from new theories about illness but from travel. Columbus's arrival in the Americas in 1492 eventually brought aloes, quinine, guaiacum (for syphilis), coca and tobacco (originally thought to be of high medicinal value, perhaps because of its use by native Americans). With the successful navigation of the route to the Far East in 1498 came rhubarb from India, senna from Africa and camphor from Japan. These and many other plants were cultivated in the botanic gardens of Renaissance Europe.

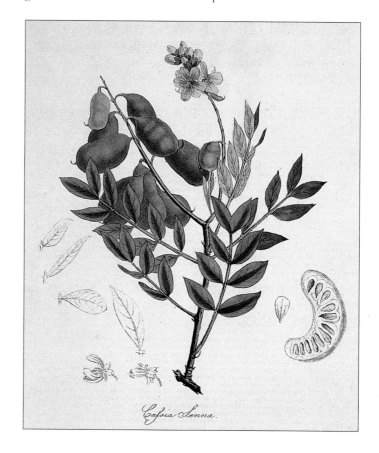

Cassia senna produces the laxative 'senna pods'. The species *was introduced to Europe from Africa.*

Acupuncture and the Chinese Pharmacopoeia

The Chinese, in common with the ancient Greeks and Romans, have a history of linking health with divine influence. They also have a very solid tradition of plant-based medicine dating from the first and second centuries BC when the delightfully named *Pharmacopoeia of the Heavenly Husbandman* listed over 300 drugs. From the sixth century BC physicians had used *The Yellow Emperor's Manual of Corporeal Medicine* and by the time of the Ming Dynasty (1368–1644) their art had developed to a high point. Thereafter, medical practice became divided into the philosophical and the practical, the latter becoming increasingly superstitious until the arrival of communism. Much of the treatment was nevertheless plant based, perhaps influenced by the Taoist tradition of venerating nature by observation.

In parallel with the use of drugs was an interest in massage, gymnastics and acupuncture. Acupuncture was first used in about 500 BC and, although temporarily banned in 1822, is still used extensively in modern China's system of devolved health care. Acupuncture involves the insertion of fine needles into the body at certain defined points that are said to be joined by invisible meridians (the twelve Ching) and two auxiliary tracts (Ho). Energy (Chi) passes along these tracts and the treatment by needles aims to restore the flow if it has become blocked or disrupted. Acupuncturists use plants as well, particularly where disease is severe, by burning small cones of powdered *Artemisia vulgaris* leaves (moxa) for precise lengths of time at specific points around the body. This technique is called moxibustion and was also used in the Japanese system of traditional medicine (Kampo) at least until the adoption of Western medical practice in Japan from the 1870s onwards.

ABOVE RIGHT: *Some Chinese acupuncturists burn* Artemisia vulgaris *at defined points on the body to heal severe disease.*
RIGHT: *Modern Chinese medicine is known for its use of 'barefoot doctors', men or women with three to six months' training who operate as community-based paramedics.*

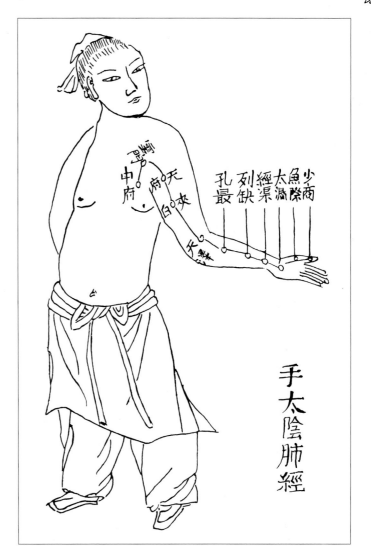

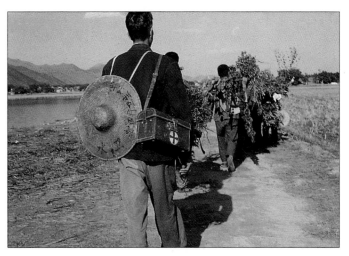

FOLK MEDICINE

There are many traditions of healing from around the world that run parallel to the type of medicine practised in the West. One of the most ancient is the Indian Ayurvedic system, which is still common at a community level in India. In Africa, the Americas, and in Australia and New Zealand, the indigenous peoples have their own medicinal practices using plants. Their ideas about healing are deeply rooted in their culture and traditions. Some have used plant drugs that have subsequently been adopted by Western medicine and double-blind tested for efficacy.

Indian Ayurvedic healing

Of all the ancient systems of medicine the one closest to the Aristotelian tradition of humours is Indian. 'Ayurveda' in Sanskrit means 'the science of life' or 'the science of (living to a ripe) age' and was dominant in the Indian sub-continent from 1500 BC until the tenth century AD. Ayurvedic doctors believe that there are seven 'dhatus' or elements (food juices, flesh, blood, fat, bones, marrow and semen) in the body and three 'tridosa' or humours (wind, bile and phlegm). In the body of a healthy person there is a good balance between the dhatus and the tridosa, which may be affected by the constitution you inherit. The principal Ayurvedic texts (the *Caralea Samhita* and the *Susruta Samhita*) date from 200 BC to AD 200 and include over 700 useful herbs classified by their action on the dhatus and tridosa, or by their effects on the patient. The tradition also stresses the need to collect the plant drugs in the right way, at the right season and from the right soil. The purity of the doctor and the way the drugs are stored are considered important, as is the patient's diet.

Today, Ayurveda is encouraged by the Indian government as an inexpensive alternative to expensive Western drugs. It is widely practised in Sri Lanka where many also believe that the humoral balance can be disturbed by demons

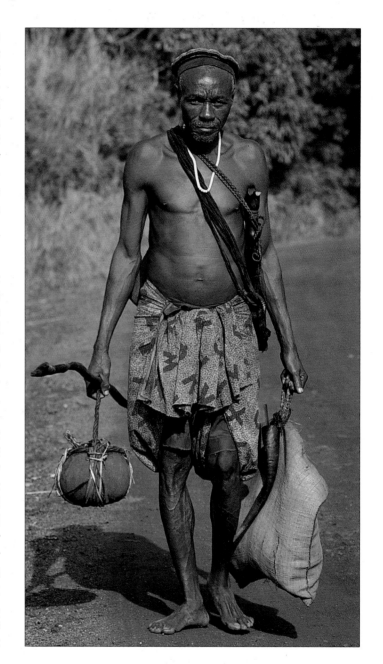

Most traditions of folk medicine around the world are rooted in the spiritual traditions of their culture which determine the causes of ill-health. Healers like this tribal doctor from Cameroon work with these beliefs using local plant and animal products which they carry to their patients.

who need to be exorcized. In Britain, Ayurveda is used by Asian communities and there is now an Ayurvedic Company of Great Britain working in association with a pharmacy in Coimbatore, southern India, that manages two therapy centres. Much of the therapy consists in the use of herbal oils that are employed in massage and in diet control; and it is claimed to be particularly effective in treating rheumatic diseases. Ayurveda has been criticized, however, for the inclusion of heavy metals in its medicines, which are now known to be toxic, especially to children.

African traditions

Most traditional African cultures believe that disease is caused by the malevolence of witches, sorcerers or evil ancestors, and medicinal healers are therefore a spiritual focus in the community. Disease is avoided by observing taboos, wearing amulets, giving offerings to beneficent ancestors or by ritual dancing. This spiritual approach is backed up by the use of the local flora by herbalists, although the herbal drugs are often thought to be more effective when used in conjunction with charms and chants. Local markets are often rich in medicinal plants that are either cultivated or plucked from the wild. South Africa has a particularly strong herbal tradition working alongside the Western medicine of the white population.

North American medicine

North American Indians have developed very distinct theories as to the spiritual causes of disease. Illness is thought to result from 'soul loss' where the soul has been kidnapped by a ghost or an enemy, by the intrusion of an object into the body through sorcery or by the breaking of a strongly held taboo.

The practice of the medicine man relates to the plant world in several ways. Some tribes believe that spirits inspire the healer to know which curative plants to use, others that a plant is protected by the spirit that has endowed it with medicinal properties. Offerings are often left to these spirits when the drug plant is picked. Healing is indicated by the return of the soul or by the

medicine man claiming to produce the 'extracted object'. Massage and ritual 'sweat baths' are also used in the healing process.

Drugs of the ancient American civilizations

In Mexico the ancient civilizations of the Mayas and the Aztecs had a strong social hierarchy with astrologer-diviners serving the medicinal needs of the nobility and herbalists those of the majority of the people. The Incas of Peru had similar beliefs to the North American Indian tribes and used plants that are well known today, including curare for digestive diseases. Cocaine was used ritualistically by healers; and quinine was known to be useful against fever long before it was discovered by the Jesuits, although the explanation of its action – that the disease-causing spirit could not bear its bitterness – was peculiarly Indian. Tobacco was a common drug used throughout the Americas; it was deified in Mexico, used as a sedative in Peru, and played a part in much of North American Indian life as a social ritual.

Aboriginal and Maori traditions

The Australian Aborigines similarly believe that illness is caused by sorcery, particularly by object intrusions. The tribal elders, in contact with their Dreaming, would claim to extract the object. Medicinal plants were, and still are, used. Anyone who has ever had a pre-med injection before an anaesthetic for surgery will have received a drug called hyoscine commercially cropped from *Duboisia myoporoides*, a medicinal plant well known to the Aborigines.

The Maoris are unique in having made very little use of plants before the arrival of European settlers. Their culture stressed the avoidance of disease by appeasing their ancestors, observing taboos and deflecting the wrath of their gods. Ill people would often move away from the area, or were even abandoned to their fate. Experimentation with their own flora was a response to seeing white settlers use herbal remedies, and became more urgent as the Maoris began to contract the diseases the settlers brought with them.

THE PHYSIC GARDEN TRADITION

○

The earliest moves towards the concept of a botanic garden began in the ancient Egyptian temple gardens at least 1000 years BC where known medicinal plants were grown. The Greeks developed botany as a philosophical study before the time of Christ and in China the reigning Emperors became some of the earliest plant collectors.

In Europe, however, it was in monasteries from the sixth century AD onwards that medicinal gardens became standard, and were sited next to the infirmary. Botany was firmly wedded to medicine and, with the foundation of the early universities in the Renaissance, the professors of the one discipline were usually the professors of the other. Still paying respect to the ideas of Swiss physician Paracelsus and Greek botanist and physician Dioscorides, plants were seen as being present on Earth for their healing benefit, known or potential. They were grown in 'physick' gardens, to serve the physician's requirements for existing or newly introduced raw materials in the healing arts and to teach medical students to distinguish between what would cure rather than kill their patients. There was no concept of botany as a systematic discipline in its own right, which is fundamental to the idea of a modern botanic garden which developed later in the eighteenth and nineteenth centuries with the introduction of new taxonomic systems.

A Victorian artist's impression of apothecaries discussing their trade in plant drugs at the Chelsea Physic Garden.

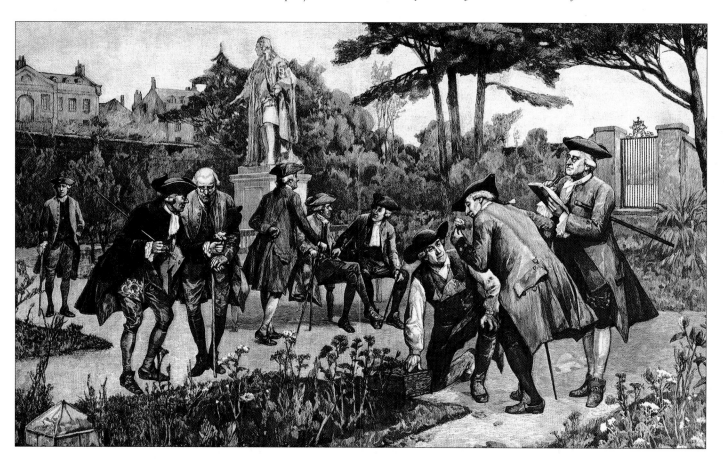

Early physic gardens

All the early physic gardens were products of the Italian Renaissance, first in Pisa in 1543 (which is still open to the public, though a weed-strewn relic of its former self) and some years later in Padua (1545) and Florence (1550). Other countries followed suit with gardens at Leipzig (1580), Heidelburg (1593), Paris (1635) and Uppsala (1665), and also at Leiden (1587) where a charming re-creation of the original 'Hortus Clusianus' has recently been completed, along with its trellis and treillage and raised beds. Crushed-shell paths have been used in a delightful (but not completely authentic) touch.

In Britain there were some private physic gardens belonging to clerics such as that of William Turner, Dean of Wells Cathedral. The first university garden was at Oxford, founded in 1621 as the Oxford Physic Garden and retaining this name until 1840, a period when medical botany was in disfavour compared to the rising independent science of systematic and observational botany. Edinburgh's garden was founded in 1656 to service the teaching of both surgeons and apothecaries (often unhappy bedfellows), and in London the Chelsea Physic Garden was founded in 1673 for the apprentices of the Society of Apothecaries, the physicians staying aloof. The Society were strained by the loss of their Livery Hall in Blackfriars in the Great Fire of London in 1666 but supported the Garden until 1899 and still fund the production of its annual seed list.

These early gardens were generally walled against wind and marauders and laid out formally. The Chelsea Physic Garden originally ran down to the river (until the building of the Embankment in the 1870s) so as to ease the transport of the apprentices by barge during their seven years' training. It is interesting that practically all botanic gardens started as physic gardens; even the Royal Botanic Gardens, Kew (started by William Aiton after training under Philip Miller at Chelsea), was established as 'Princess Augusta's Physic Garden'. Today, of all the ancient gardens in Britain, it is Chelsea alone that retains its origi-

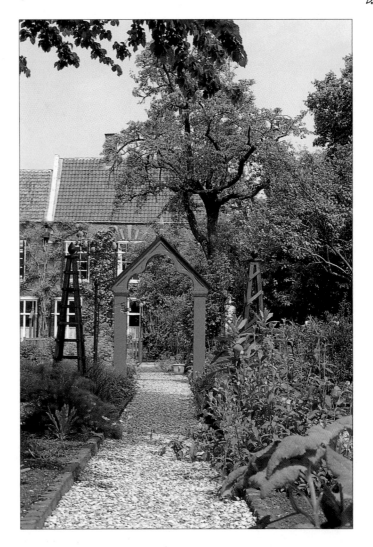

The 'Hortus Clusianus' or Clusius Garden at the Leiden Botanic Garden in Holland is a meticulous re-creation of Clusius's original physic garden. Bounded by the walls of buildings, it gives an accurate impression of the intimacy of many of these early formal gardens, and is totally authentic apart from the use of crushed shell for the paths.

nal title. There is, however, a move to create or restore physic gardens, particularly in the United States under the aegis of the American Herb Society, for example at Morristown, New Jersey and Yellow Springs, Pennsylvania. In Britain modern physic gardens with an educational and display purpose can be seen at Petersfield in Hampshire and at Hitchin in Hertfordshire.

THE APOTHECARIES' GARDEN OF SIMPLES

John Evelyn, the seventeenth-century diarist, called the Chelsea Physic Garden the Apothecaries' Garden of Simples. This was a reference to the medicinal function of the Garden for a 'simple' was a single medicinal plant, one of many ingredients from which an apothecary would produce a compound medicine.

The herbals of the time showed that nearly every plant was assumed to have some medicinal use. This was partly due to the long-held belief in the 'Doctrine of Signatures' whereby it was thought that the appearance of a plant gave a sign or indication of the type of disease it would cure. With the development of medical science this idea fell out of favour by the mid-seventeenth century. There was, however, a continuing belief in the potential of plants to cure if only the right plant could be matched with the right disorder.

The cultivation of medicinal plants

One of the earliest medicinal plants cultivated in the stove glasshouses at Chelsea was Jesuits' Bark *Cinchona* species, introduced from South America,

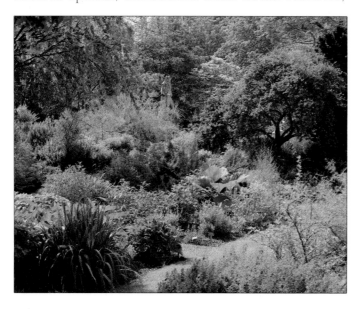

Sir Hans Sloane, who granted land for Chelsea Physic Garden.

from which we obtain quinine, the main drug used to combat malaria in the tropics. Another was *Vinca rosea*, now known as *Catharanthus roseus* Madagascar Periwinkle, which is today the main source of alkaloids used in the treatment of leukaemia and Hodgkin's disease. Chelsea cultivated and distributed this plant to other botanic gardens after it had first been introduced via the Jardin des Plantes in Paris.

During the first century of the Garden's life, its gardener Philip Miller greatly extended its function. He became a specialist in growing a wide variety of fruits and vegetables, including melons, and through his correspondence solicited many new species, especially from the Americas. His *Gardener's Dictionary* was republished in eight editions and the Garden became famous throughout Europe. Miller's successors maintained medicinal collections, although they all had interests of their own, and inventories by some of them such as Thomas Moore, Curator 1848–87, still exist. Robert Fortune, noted plant collector and Curator at Chelsea from 1846–48, introduced tea from China to India. The transportation of young tea plants was made using a series of Wardian cases, miniature travelling glasshouses designed by Nathaniel Bagshaw Ward, an examiner of the apothecary students at the Garden.

Although the Garden was secure in its lease of land under the terms of its benefactor Sir Hans Sloane, for many years the Society of Apothecaries found the annual running costs beyond its means. Eventually, in 1899, the Society relinquished the Garden to the Trustees of the London Parochial Charities who ran it as a research resource for various London colleges.

The Chelsea Physic Garden today

The Society of Apothecaries retains links with the Garden in funding the annual exchange of seeds with other botanic gardens worldwide, and a further legacy remains in its handsome crest on the

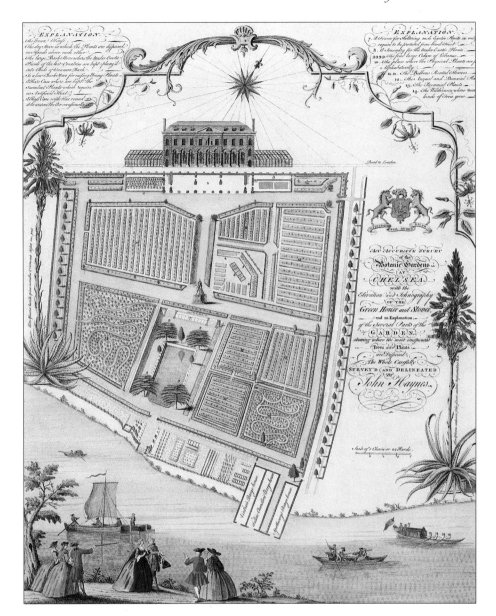

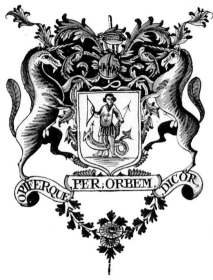

ABOVE: *Coat of arms of the Worshipful Society of Apothecaries of London from a tile. Tiles were used to prepare medicines on.*

LEFT: *The Chelsea Physic Garden was founded in 1673 by the Worshipful Society of Apothecaries of London as a place of instruction for their own apprentices, its riverside location providing easy access by barge from the City of London. This view of the garden was drawn in 1751 and shows its carefully planned layout, with individual plots for the growth and study of particular plant species.*

Embankment Gates and in the old Students' Bell inside the Swan Walk Gate. Today, the garden is run by its own body of Trustees. It has maintained a research link with Glaxo Group Research Limited since 1989, providing dried specimens in their search for new medicines from plants. As part of its educational work the Garden maintains a 'Medicinal Walk' that displays the history of plant medicine from Dioscorides and the 'Doctrine of Signatures', onwards. There is a bed displaying all the major drug plants in use today, and a selection of tropical medicinal plants is cultivated in the glasshouse range. There is also a garden of world medicine, where ethnomedical plants (used, for example, by the Chinese and North American Indians) are grown. Although the garden has other functions, including research, conservation, education and the provision of an amenity, it remains linked to the display and continuing research of medicinal plants and Chelsea is the only early Garden to retain its original title of Physic Garden.

MEDICINAL HERBS AND HERBALISM

Herbalism has its origins in an age-old basic belief that plants exist to provide remedies for the body's ills.

In medieval times, and up until the seventeenth century, the knowledge and lore of herbs was written down in herbals. These books were sometimes illustrated with woodcuts, often done by monks who simply copied the illustrations of plants from their forebears until they became either crudely diagrammatic or totally fanciful. With the Renaissance, however, came an interest in observing and drawing real plants from nature and some of the herbals of Otto Brunfels and Leonard Fuchs, for example, are absolute gems of plant portraiture. In England the most famous herbals were those of John Gerard and Nicholas Culpeper, the name of the latter commemorated in one of Britain's most successful chains of modern herbal retailers.

Nevertheless, this written tradition should not blind us to the fact that a lot of knowledge was passed on from generation to generation by word of mouth. Generally, especially in medieval times, women were the 'herb gatherers' and it was the lower classes of society who relied on their wares. Educated and wealthier people preferred to be treated with the mineral-based drugs of the physicians. By the eighteenth century herbalism had lost its popularity, although it remained in practice by the rural poor and also in colonial America and New Zealand.

In 1864 the National Association of Medical Herbalists was formed in Britain. This organization still exists (as the National Institute of Medical Herbalists) and, with over 300 members in its own country, is the oldest such association.

Herbalism today

The modern herbalist uses a rich variety of vegetable matter for healing purposes, not just the culinary and aromatic 'herbs' with which we are familiar in the kitchen. About 85 per cent of the global population still relies on herbalism for its basic health care. This is not to say that all herbal remedies are proven, however, nor to say that all 'natural' plant remedies are gentle and harmless; after all, some of the most deadly poisons come from plants.

Sometimes herbal remedies have been taken up by orthodox Western medicine, tested and been proved effective according to double-blind testing. An example is ginger, which contains a substance that counters motion sickness more effectively than synthetic drugs.

There remains, however, a basic conflict between the *theory* that underlies herbalism and that of orthodox medicine. The herbalist believes in the healing properties of the whole plant and rejects the isolation of a chemical principle from it. These properties work together to heal, which is why herbalism is considered a holistic therapy. Orthodox medicine rejects this as a theory with no firm scientific evidence and pharmaceutical companies continue to screen for active chemical principles within plants, often synthesizing them chemically for prescription as drugs. A biochemist once suggested to me that these opposing views could be reconciled by the notion that chemicals within the plant act together (synergistically) to create the healing effect. The main point, though, is that the herbalist trusts the effect of the plant itself rather than chemistry. This approach appeals to many people because they have experienced side effects from synthetic drugs or because they wish to return to a type of healing that seems closer to nature.

Herbalists generally prescribe medicines in the form of alcohol-based tinctures, and only after a long diagnostic discussion with the patient to ascertain his or her emotional and psychological state and any other factors that may affect the holistic process. In this regard herbalists are similar to homoeopaths (see page 22) in their consultation procedure.

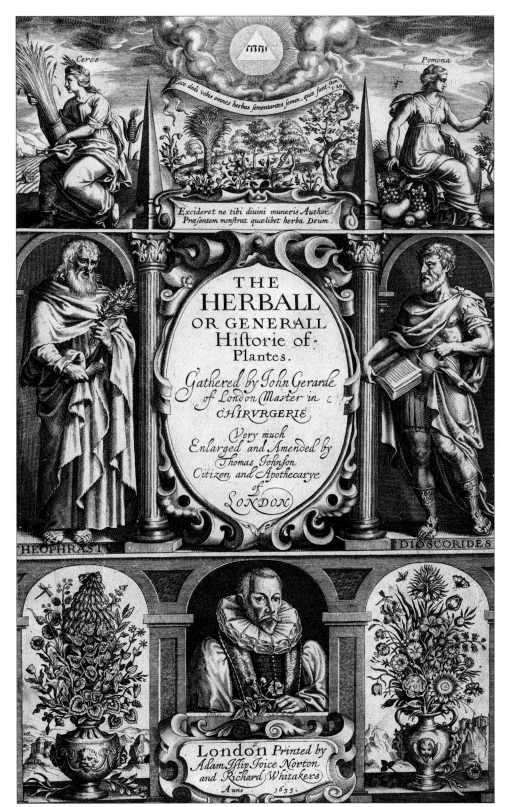

It is generally recognized that John Gerard's Herball was a compilation of the work of earlier herbalists. The beautiful frontispiece of the 1633 edition, shown here, includes portraits of Dioscorides and Theophrastus, two of the most significant Greek physicians who worked with plants, as well as Gerard himself. Gerard's Herball became the best known herbal in Britain, Nicholas Culpeper's The English Physician following in 1653. Such herbals were intended as practical handbooks to assist in the correct identification and use of plants in 'chirurgerie', an alternative name for 'surgery'.

HOMOEOPATHIC NATURAL CURES

Homoeopathy is a system of healing in which like is treated with like, a principle known to the Greek physician Hippocrates in the fifth century BC but not developed until the early nineteenth century in Germany. Its chief proponent was Dr Samuel Hahnemann, who was concerned at the harsh medical approaches of the time in which blood-letting and the use of arsenic were common. He coined the name 'homoeopathy' for the new method from the Greek *homoios* meaning 'like' as opposed to conventional or 'allopathic' medicine that used drugs to fight against disease. At the heart of the system is a differing approach to the meaning of medical symptoms. Orthodox medicine maintains that these result from the disease and need to be suppressed. Homoeopaths claim that the symptoms express the body's attempt to heal itself and, indeed, may need to be encouraged.

In homoeopathy, substances that produce the same symptoms as those of the disease itself are used as cures. Not all of these are plant based – almost half of the major cures derive from vegetable matter, the rest being mineral salts, or animal or other biological materials. However, Hahnemann is said to have been led to his ideas by observing how a plant (cinchona bark) produced fever in a healthy person, yet cured malaria.

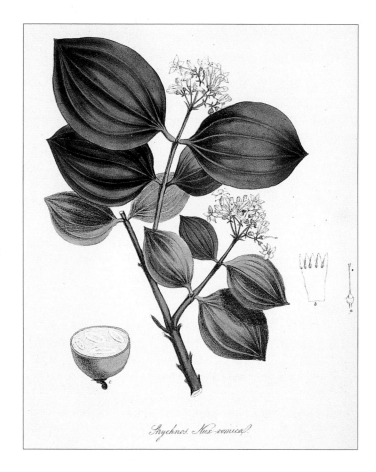

Strychnos *is toxic unless prepared homoeopathically.*

How does homoeopathy 'work'?

Homoeopathy qualifies as a 'holistic' therapy because it concentrates on all the facets of a person – spiritual, mental and emotional as well as physical. Each of these facets can affect the progress of a disease and each needs to be assessed before an appropriate treatment can be selected. New patients often find it strange to have their appearance, reactions, beliefs and fears assessed as well as their symptoms! The aim is to restore health by restoring balance so that the body can heal itself, thus healing the person and not treating the disease. In a complex or prolonged cure, homoeopaths believe that the symptoms of a disease may worsen before they are relieved and that previous symptoms may resurface before disappearing. Symptoms can also 'move' about the body in the process of healing, from internal organs to more superficial sites.

Probably the most controversial side of homoeopathy is the belief that the remedies are made more potent by extreme dilution, while also being made more safe. Allopathic doctors often say that the dilution is so great that scarcely a molecule of the original substance can remain. Homoeopaths respond that they do not know *how* their system works, but that they *see* that it does.

PLANT REMEDIES USED IN HOMOEOPATHY

Name Botanical; Common; Homoeopathic	Physical symptoms	Emotional state
Aconitum napellus; Aconite; Aconite	Sudden chill, dry cough, sore throat following chill, fever with thirst, intense pain, motion sickness, insomnia.	Bereavement or grief, anxiety, fear, restlessness, panic attacks.
Actaea spicata; Baneberry; Actaea	Headache, neuralgia, muscle strain, rheumatic stiffness in upper body.	Depression, confusion.
Arnica montana; Arnica; Arnica	Bruises, sprains, muscle strain, gout, rheumatism.	Overtiredness, sensitivity to being touched.
Atropa belladonna; Deadly Nightshade; Belladonna	Swelling of joints, neuralgia, earache, throbbing headache, dry cough, motion sickness and vertigo, acne, cystitis, colic, insomnia.	Lively cheerful disposition.
Bryonia alba; White Bryony; Bryonia	Chesty colds, pleurisy, dry cough, dry lips, thirst, colic, arthritis.	Irritable.
†*Cephaelis (Psychotria) ipecacuanha;* Ipecacuanha; Ipecacuanha	Nausea, sickness, bronchitis, breathlessness.	–
Drosera rotundifolia; Sundew; Drosera	Coughs, sickness, laryngitis, vertigo.	–
Euphrasia officinalis; Eyebright; Euphrasia	Streaming colds, conjunctivitis, sensitivity to strong light, hayfever, eyestrain.	–
†*Gelsemium sempervirens;* Carolina Jasmine; Gelsemium	Influenza and its symptoms, absence of thirst with fever, delirium, difficulty in swallowing.	Nervous excitability, worry, phobic personality.
Hamamelis virginiana; Witch Hazel; Hamamelis	Varicose veins, nosebleeds, bleeding piles, tired and sore limbs, chilblains.	–
Hypericum perforatum; St John's Wort; Hypericum	Painful wounds, injuries from falls, injured fingers and toes, piles, insect bites.	–
Lycopodium clavatum; Club Moss; Lycopodium	Hunger cravings, especially for sweet things, stomach irritability, cystitis, menstrual problems, premature baldness and greying.	Irritability, fear of failure, intenseness and insecurity, unsociability.
Pulsatilla pratensis spp. *nigricans;* Pulsatilla; Pulsatilla	Catarrh, hayfever, styes, period pain or irregularity, premenstrual tension, cystitis, acne, tinnitus, arthritis, dry mouth.	Affectionate, responsive, weepy.
Ruta graveolens; Rue; Ruta graveolens	Fractures, sprains, dislocations, rheumatism, arthritis, eye strain, nettle rash.	–
●†*Strychnos nux-vomica;* Nux Vomica; Nux Vomica	Nervous indigestion, liverishness, constipation, piles, premenstrual tension.	Impatience, irritability, anxiousness.
Thuja occidentalis; White Cedar; Thuja	Warts, styes, frequent urination, headaches.	Strong, stubborn and opinionated.
●*Toxicodendron radicans;* Poison Ivy; Rhus toxicodendron	Strains and sprains, sciatica, rheumatism, lumbago, arthritis, shingles, thirst, cold sores.	Restlessness.

KEY: * easily cultivated in gardens with temperate climates   † tropical species   ● not recommended for cultivation

SAVING THE WORLD'S FLORA
○

In the 1980s the growing awareness of threat to the natural environment by the actions of human beings became termed a 'green consciousness'. Nature was no longer seen as a vast system that could remain largely unaffected by what we do. Increasing evidence has shown the destruction of the protective ozone layer by chlorofluorocarbons, along with worrying indications of climate change and the pollution of groundwater. Such problems, as well as events such as nuclear accidents, have forced us to accept responsibility for wise management of the planet.

One of our greatest losses has been the sense of the 'wild' which Thoreau saw as being essential to the health of the human spirit. Overpopulation and an increase in travel have effectively shrunk the planet so that it becomes increasingly difficult to 'go where no man has gone before'. In towns and cities people try to reconnect with the natural world in their gardens.

Conservation and medicines

The battle to conserve plants relates to the healing arts in several ways. The World Wide Fund for Nature estimated that over a quarter of prescriptions dispensed in the USA between 1959 and 1980 contained a principal ingredient derived from a plant. On a world scale they estimated that 85 per cent of drugs are *in some way* linked to a plant source. The reduction in the variety of plants as some species become extinct threatens to limit the discovery of possible future medicines. Several of our most important drugs are derived from tropical rainforest plants, including contraceptive steroids from *Dioscorea* species, muscle relaxants from curare, and pilocarpine and physostigmine for the treatment of glaucoma from *Pilocarpus* and *Physostigma*. The current loss of rainforest on a massive scale wipes out species before there has been a chance to screen them for medicinal value. In Amazonia, for example, only 1 per cent of the flora has been screened so far. The disturbance of indigenous peoples, lack of respect for their way of life and their annihilation through introduced diseases also takes away their experience of the value of the flora. Yet these people depend on the plants of the forest and desert for natural remedies and they have a vast knowledge, passed on orally from generation to generation. Tropical forests contain half the world's total plant species in only 7 per cent of the land surface of the globe. This is why conservation in the tropics and respect for the knowledge of indigenous peoples is such a key concern.

The World Health Organization has recently developed a Traditional Medicine Programme with the aim of encouraging member states to create national inventories of their medicinal plants, and develop methods of testing their efficacy and conserving their stocks. For many countries this means giving value to folk medicine at primary care level and in rural areas.

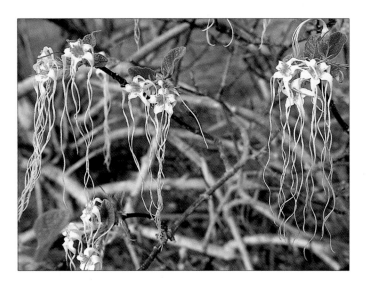

LEFT: Strophanthus *is used as arrow poison by African bushmen. Its action has been used in cardiac drug research.*
RIGHT: *Preparing curare as an arrow poison in Colombia. Tubocurarine and other synthetic derivatives are used surgically as muscle relaxants.*

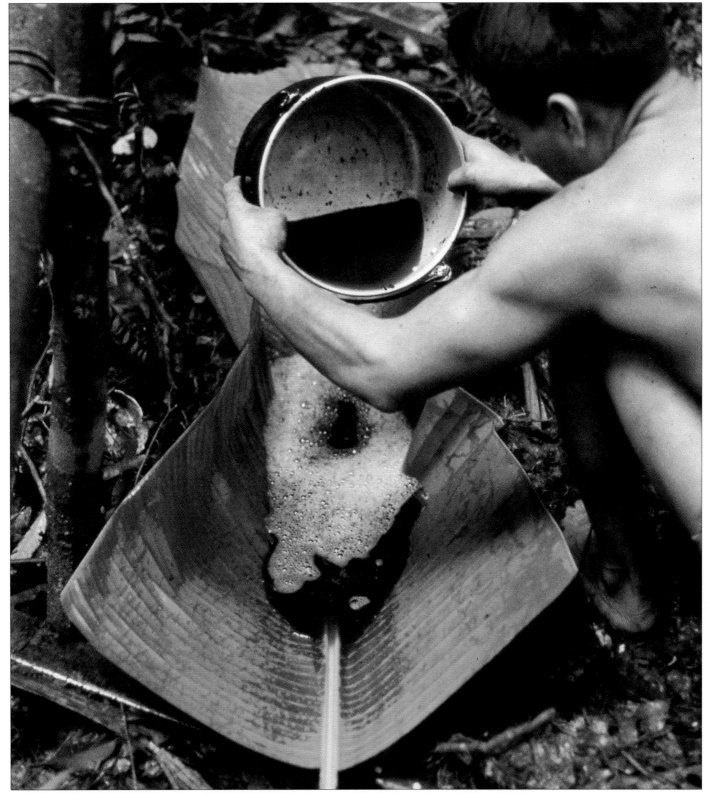

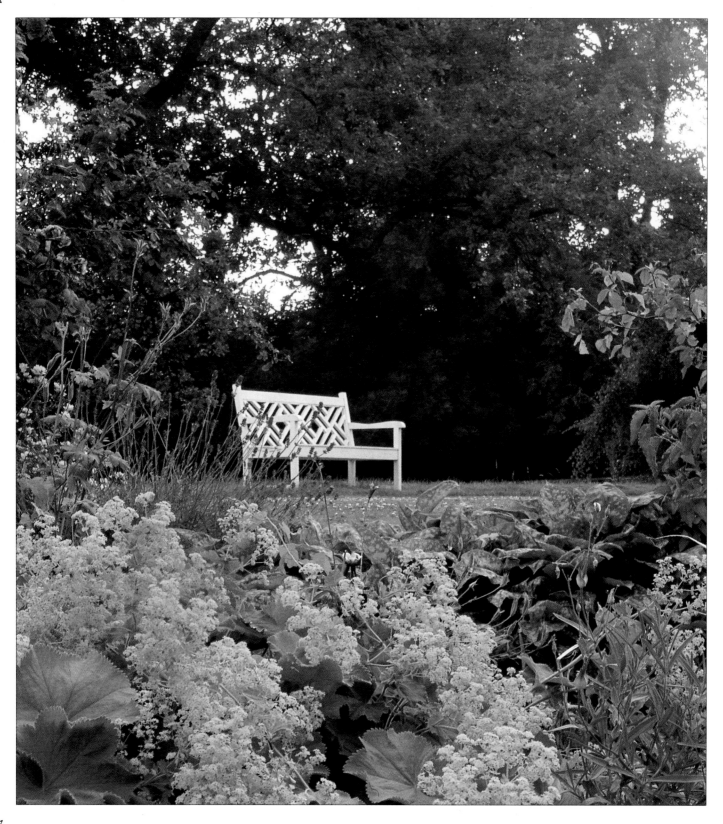

STRESS: A HIDDEN KILLER?

The idea that stress can cause disease or make it worse is comparatively recent. It is also medically controversial and considered by some to be scientifically unproven. With the 'green movement', research into environmental stress in the form of pollution has come to the fore, and we are also looking carefully at our urban surroundings, lifestyles and patterns of work. The general assumption is that life has become more stressful, involving constant changes to which we must adapt and which we often experience as a sense of loss. It is this sort of stress (as opposed to mere pressure) that is thought to predispose a person to disease by making him or her vulnerable, lowering the body's resistance to infection.

How this happens is of interest to immunologists and virologists, particularly those involved in work on cancer therapy and research into Acquired Immune Deficiency Syndrome (AIDS). Psychoneuroimmunology is the new science of looking at the relationship between stress, personality type and immune function. It is highly controversial, particularly in the field of cancer therapy where the concept of the 'cancer-prone personality' (inhibited in self-expression) is now considered unhelpful in seeming to 'blame' the patient, furthering feelings of anxiety and guilt.

Natural 'cures' for stress-related illness

Patients who suffer from AIDS are generally advised to live a life as free of stress as possible. Research is continuing and is likely to be even more important as immune deficiency diseases increase. Anything that promises hope of remission in AIDS is being examined, including plants with a reputation for boosting the immune system. One of the most recently studied is

Gardens can be 'stress-free zones' where people can relax alone or in company as preferred. Contact with the natural world can remind us of inner growth and change.

castanospermine, an extract of the Queensland Chestnut *Castanospermum australe*, which appears to inhibit virus replication.

It is known that the recently bereaved are more likely to be hospitalized with illness than control groups who have not experienced such trauma. As a society, we in the West are not good at coping with death – or with the many smaller losses we suffer, such as loss of job, of status, or of a familiar way of life – and this is not helped by traditional medical attitudes that pay more attention to disease patterns than to the emotional needs of the patient, often under the demands of time and financial stringency.

So-called 'holistic' therapies, such as herbalism and homoeopathy, consider the entire make-up of the individual, both physical (soma) and emotional (psyche). This seems sensible in that sufferers themselves are frequently aware that under stress their condition worsens. Orthodox doctors often have little time to concern themselves with the possible psychological causes of illness, and the term 'psychosomatic' may be used dismissively with the implication that symptoms are not 'real' rather than genuine emotional stress converted into a physical symptom. This perhaps explains some of the interest in alternative medicines where the approach does not strictly divide mind and body. It may also explain why some people under stress actually have physical symptoms: they can go to the doctor for help only with a physical illness and so they produce one so that it can be dealt with!

Stressed individuals often turn to the natural world for relief. Whether our working day is regimented by machinery, meetings or deadlines we all find a haven in the natural growth rhythms of a garden in the peace of evening. We should trust this response and recognize it as healing. It has been shown quite conclusively that hospital patients recover more quickly when they have a view of a garden.

GAIA: A NEW WORLD VIEW

The theory of Gaia is that the Earth, and all plant and animal life upon it, is one vast living organism, the name being derived from the ancient Greek for Mother Earth. This theory was first developed by a British scientist, James Lovelock, in the late 1970s and published as *Gaia: a New Look at Life on Earth*. Further developing and defending the theory in *The Ages of Gaia: A Biography of Our Living Earth*, Lovelock argues that the planet itself is alive in the sense of being a self-regulating and self-organizing system and that his analysis of this is a 'systems science'.

Paradoxically, these controversial views came not from the 'green movement' as such but from the highly technological world of space research, particularly from NASA's work in searching for life elsewhere in the universe. The breathtakingly beautiful views of planet Earth seen for the first time by orbiting astronauts gave many scientists a new perspective, literally a new world view, and a curiosity about the systems that support life. Whereas ecologists tended to look at the interdependence of a plant and animal ecosystem, Lovelock looked at the interregulation of all ecosystems on a global scale. Ecology expanded into a new science of 'geophysiology' or the study of interconnection and regulation between all ecosystems. These ideas are not new, as Lovelock freely admits. James Hutton in 1785 claimed that the earth is a superorganism and that some of its cycling (for example, of water, and of mineral nutrients) could be compared to the circulation of the blood. The theory is also close to some of the medieval ideas about the microcosm and macrocosm, to Renaissance ideas that considered man and planet as machines working in conjunction and even to the 'astrological' medicine of Nicholas Culpeper that related the movement of the planets to symptoms in the body (see page 12).

For me, the essential point about the work of Lovelock, is that it humbles human beings. In Gaia, human beings are not the lords of creation, with dominion over plant and animal life. Humanity is simply one species among many, not there to exploit, or even to steward other life forms, and we are ultimately expendable if our abuse of the environment threatens the stability of the Gaian system as a whole.

Several of the Gaian theorists are biologists or microbiologists who write knowledgeably about plant life from its most primitive to its most advanced forms. However, their perspective is obviously global and for them plants are less important as sources of healing than as regulators of the water, carbon and nitrogen cycles and ultimately of the world's climate. Plants create and drive the atmosphere and are therefore part of the 'self-healing' of planet Earth itself, playing a far larger role indeed.

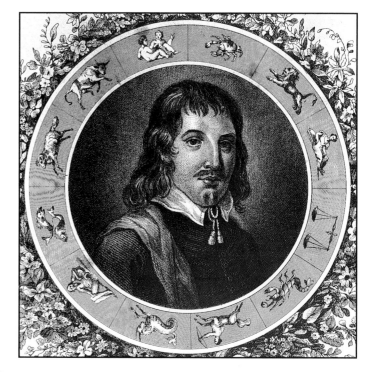

ABOVE: Nicholas Culpeper (1616–54) related plants to the astrological signs.
RIGHT: Inscrutability in a garden setting.

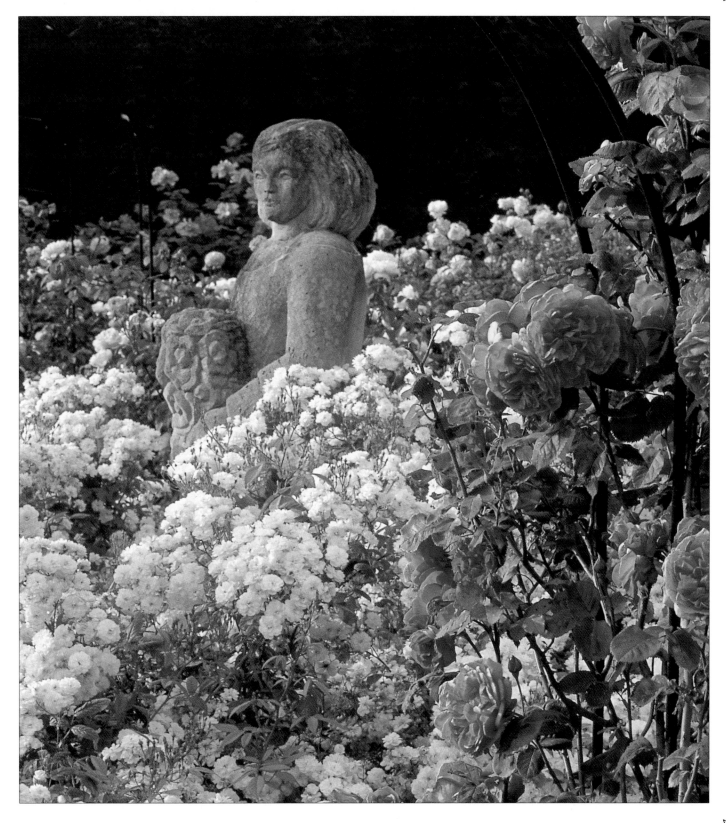

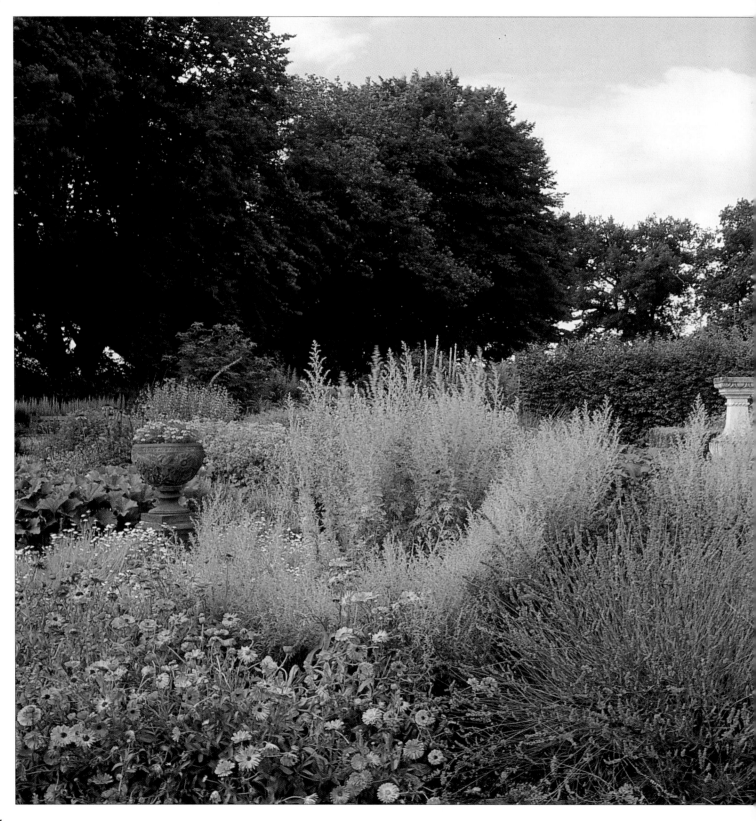

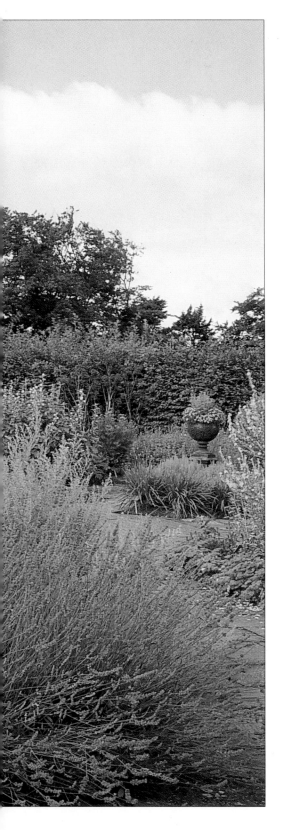

CHAPTER TWO

THE BODY PHYSICAL

○

Nature's pharmacy

There are some plants from the wide catalogue of nature's pharmacy that are easy to grow and use to treat the body's ills. Gardens can be designed around these plants like the physic gardens of old, a herbalist's retreat indeed. With today's greater knowledge of nutrition you can also include fruits and vegetables that are particularly beneficial to bodily health in the fibre, vitamins and minerals they contain.

Many of the plants that are of great importance in today's pharmaceutical industry are also very attractive as garden plants. This opens the opportunity to design an ornamental 'garden of drugs'. Whether you are interested in allopathic, homoeopathic or herbal medicine there is a medicinal garden waiting to be designed to remind you of the role plants play in the treatment of the body physical. Some key species that keep the body well are illustrated on pages 32–33.

The herb garden of the Royal Horticultural Society at Wisley, Surrey, England. The display includes Calendula, used in homoeopathy; Lavandula, used in aromatherapy; and Artemisia and Verbascum species used in herbalism.

PLANTS TO KEEP YOU WELL

○

For centuries physicians and apothecaries used plants as remedies for minor ailments and general well-being. Here is a selection for you to grow. They include plants used by herbalists and homoeopaths, and plants cropped for the pharmaceutical industry.

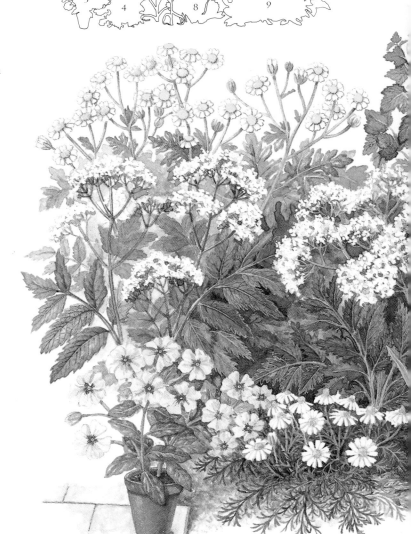

1. Feverfew *Tanacetum parthenium* is of use in the treatment of fever and headache, particularly migraine. Plant this herb in spring.

2. The herb Valerian *Valeriana officinalis* is used as a herbal and homoeopathic remedy for anxiety. Plant in spring.

3. Rosy Periwinkle *Catharanthus roseus* contains alkaloids extracted direct from the plant to treat leukaemia. Grow as a pot plant and keep it in a warm room in bright light.

4. Camomile *Chamaemelum nobile* contains oils that are useful in reducing inflammation and fevers when taken as a herbal tea. Sow outdoors in spring.

5. Garlic *Allium sativum* is a bulbous plant that contains pungent oils used against infection, in treating worms and arteriosclerosis. Plant cloves in a warm spot in spring.

6. Black Currant *Ribes nigrum* is a fruiting shrub which produces soft fruit with a high vitamin C content useful in countering infection and preventing scurvy. Plant as a bush in autumn.

7. The Opium Poppy *Papaver somniferum* is a self-seeding annual that contains morphine, the finest pain reliever, and its derivative, codeine. Sow in mid spring.

8. Meadow Saffron *Colchicum autumnale* is an autumn-flowering bulb which yields a useful remedy for gout and is of use in cancer research. Plant in late summer.

9. The Marigold *Calendula officinalis* is an annual plant and contains wound-healing substances when applied as a compress and an ointment. Sow outdoors in spring.

10. Lemon Verbena *Aloysia triphylla* is a tender shrub which contains an oil that aids digestion and reduces fever. It is best taken as an infusion. Plant in early summer against a warm, sheltered wall.

11. Fennel *Foeniculum vulgare* is a perennial herb which contains oils that are effective against gaseous indigestion, especially when the seeds are used as a tea. Sow outdoors in spring.

12. Evening Primrose *Oenothera biennis* is a biennial herb which contains acids of use in treating eczema and reputedly of use against premenstrual tension. Plant in spring.

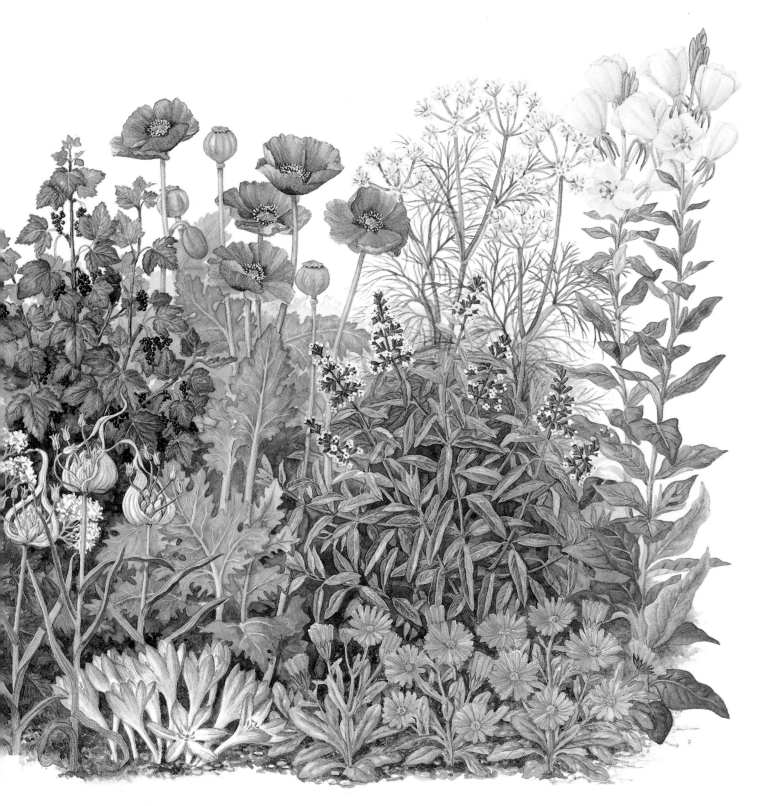

HEALTHY EATING

'You are what you eat' is a relatively new idea in the West. In fact, the entire science of nutrition and the metabolism of food in the body only developed in the West in the early twentieth century. This is late compared to other areas of the world; in India, for example, diet has always been seen as important in the ancient Ayurvedic code of healing.

In recent years there have been many debates concerning food and its effects on health. The 1980s and 90s have brought a concern with the effects of synthetic colorants and additives on health, and particularly on possible links between these and hyperactivity in children.

The diets of many Americans and Northern Europeans are currently thought to be too high in sugar, salt, saturated fats and protein, and too low in unsaturated fats, some carbohydrates and fibre, the worst items meriting the name of 'junk food'.

There is also pressure on manufacturers to produce convenience foods for quick preparation and advertisers become ever more adept at producing foods tailored to the latest 'food fad'.

The vegetarian option

One of the longest-running controversies has been the discovery of the relation between over-saturated fat and arterial disease. Studies of natural patterns of health have revealed high rates of heart disease among populations with high intakes of animal fats, which in turn has fuelled a move towards vegetarianism.

Fibre in food is now considered essential in maintaining good digestive health so there is a move towards eating more raw fruit and raw, lightly steamed or stir-fried vegetables and high-fibre cereals, a diet that is much closer to Chinese and Asian traditions.

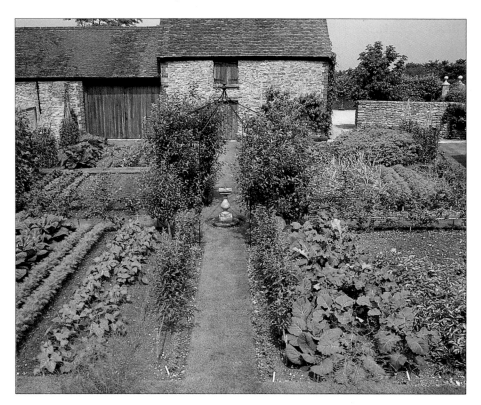

Country houses and estates would once have had a walled kitchen garden to provide fresh produce. Nowadays, many people enjoy vegetables from their own gardens or from allotment plots where they can produce fresh food with control over what pesticides, if any, they employ. There is also the pleasure of experimenting with new crops or new varieties of old ones and the physical benefit of exercise. Allotments often provide a social benefit as well – of community and competition.

Vegetarianism has also been boosted by revulsion against modern methods of factory farming of animals for meat, both on moral and health grounds. There is growing suspicion about the use of growth-boosting hormones and the residues of regular dosing with antibiotics made necessary by intensive stocking. Residues of pesticides and herbicides in fruit and vegetables and in artificially farmed fish have concerned enough people to stimulate a demand for organic produce. Many supermarkets now stock such produce which commands premium prices, and there is a health food shop catering for vegetarians in most sizeable towns.

Growing your own vegetables and fruit is an enjoyable way of producing food that is guaranteed free of harmful residues at an acceptable cost.

Macrobiotics and yin yang

Macrobiotics is the principle of applying many of the theories of oriental medicine to diet, particularly the theory of the complementary opposites yin and yang (female and male) which are thought to be present in all aspects of life to produce the balanced whole. This philosophy was one of the most important elements in the early 'natural food' movement, particularly in the belief that 'you are what you eat'.

A macrobiotic diet is primarily a vegetarian or near-vegetarian diet based on grain, and is thought to be closest to what our physiology shows we are evolved to eat. The core of such a diet is derived from grains and pulses, vegetables, seeds, nuts and a little fruit. These are all thought to be 'balanced foods'. Yang foods (such as meat, salt, eggs, fish and hard cheeses) are thought to cause disease in excess, as is excessive consumption of yin foods (such as sugar, fruit juices, dairy products, and plant products like herbs, spices and plant-derived beverages). However, you can incorporate some of these foods into your diet to balance your physical and mental health. Even the methods of preparation and cooking of foods can be classified as yin and yang, and further affect the balance of the meal, deep frying being the most yang and boiling the most yin.

A STANDARD MACROBIOTIC DIET

A macrobiotic diet is typically composed of about 73 per cent carbohydrates (from whole cereals, vegetables and pulses), 12 per cent protein (from grains, pulses, fish, nuts and seeds) and 15 per cent fat (from grain, beans, seeds and nuts). Little fruit and no sugar is consumed. The food should not be imported.

You can make a standard meal by following the proportions of ingredients in the following chart.

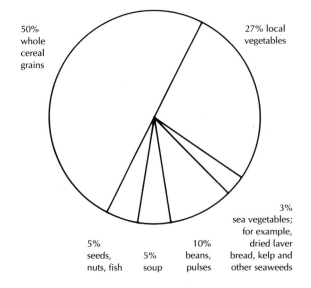

50% whole cereal grains

27% local vegetables

3% sea vegetables; for example, dried laver bread, kelp and other seaweeds

10% beans, pulses

5% soup

5% seeds, nuts, fish

Peanuts are a valuable source of protein.

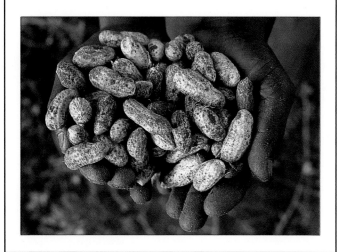

Producing the maximum crop in a small space is a frequent requirement in town gardens. Growing runner beans on a wigwam of canes is the best way of maximizing the yields of this crop. Pests can be deterred by 'companion planting'. In this case the pungent foliage of French Marigolds is thought to deter blackfly attack. Runner beans need high soil fertility and ample moisture, so good soil preparation is important.

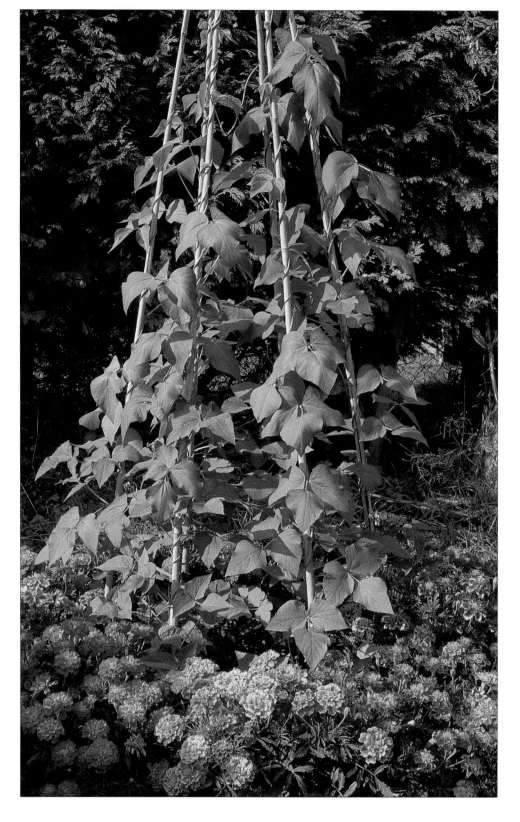

ORGANIC GARDENING

○

Growing produce that is free of pesticides and herbicides involves managing your garden organically, and as an organic gardener you have a different view of the soil from that of the gardener who depends on chemical fertilizers. The soil is not a mere carrier of chemicals, rather it is a complex structure that needs proper husbandry and respect for its physical properties.

Looking after the soil

You can maintain a good soil structure by adding plenty of organic matter such as garden compost or well-rotted farmyard manure. (How to make compost is described on page 38.) This helps to aerate the soil, assisting both drainage and moisture retention at the same time. Never walk on your soil when it is wet or you will cause damage by compacting it, forcing out the air and breaking down its structure. Adding lime or gypsum helps the structure of extremely clayey soil.

The pros and cons of digging often cause heated debate among organic gardeners. The 'no dig' school claims that digging is a totally unnatural activity and should be replaced by mulching the soil. On the other hand, anyone who has seen the rampant growth of weeds on landslides and landslips will see that plants do respond to the aeration that soil movement provides. I suggest that the answer is to know your own soil. If it is light it will probably need minimum digging and a good deal of mulching. Clay-based heavy soils are best dug or rotavated in the early autumn *before they get wet* and left rough so that frost action will provide a good tilth on the surface for spring sowing direct into the ground.

Garden compost

Good composting should be at the heart of any organic gardening system, and is a simple way of recycling the waste that a garden produces. Garden compost improves the structure of the soil, so assisting root growth and good drainage. It helps prevent the soil becoming compacted and provides nourishment for the plants. If applied as a mulch to *moist* soil, compost will also suppress weeds as well as retaining moisture.

Potting compost

It is important not to confuse the two terms 'garden compost' and 'potting compost'. Potting compost is used for potting plants and can be bought from any garden centre. It consists of ingredients that are sterile so as not to introduce bacterial and fungal diseases to seedlings and young plants. Potting composts are usually made up of a mixture of sterilized loam, grit or perlite and a dressing of fertilizers and trace elements. In Britain peat-based composts have generally been replaced by coconut fibre (coir) based composts to conserve the dwindling peat lands of Britain and Ireland, many of which have been designated Sites of Special Scientific Interest.

Dealing with weeds

If you garden organically you cannot use synthetic chemicals to kill existing weeds or to prevent weeds germinating. Weedkillers were developed mainly to help farmers faced with lack of labouring help as people left the land to work in urban areas. So be prepared to put more of your own labour into dealing with weeds organically! This can be a pleasure in itself if you enjoy gardening.

You should never let ground stand bare. Water it well and cover the surface with a 7.5cm (3in) layer of organic matter to stop weeds germinating. If ground does have to stand bare for some reason, sow it with a proprietary 'green' manure. Dig this in when it has matured.

Never let a weed produce seed. The old adage 'one year's seed means seven years' weeds' is very true. Do not dig or disturb the soil more than you must during the growing season as this will bring up more weed seed. Be prepared to work with the weather; hoeing off weeds in hot sunshine will

HOW TO MAKE GARDEN COMPOST

It is not difficult to make compost provided some simple principles are followed.

Choose a place out of sight of the rest of the garden but with good access for barrows. Use wood to construct two bins side by side, each measuring at least 1 metre (3 ft) cubed. Make the front slats removable so that you can gain access to the compost. Wood is the best material to use as it insulates well. Do not skimp on the size of the bins as you need a large volume to generate the heat necessary for decomposition and to make sure that weed seed is killed.

Each bin can be open to the soil at the bottom to allow earthworms in. They will improve both breakdown and aeration.

It is always best to make compost in one go, so you may need to store garden waste in bags or heaps until you have accumulated enough. Use just one bin to make the compost in. Put the coarsest material at the bottom to assist drainage and then build it up with layers of waste at least 15cm (6in) deep. Chop up the remaining coarse waste and allow some soil in since it adds bacteria.

Avoid adding the roots of perennial weeds. Include some sort of material such as poultry or animal manure that will accelerate decay by supplying nitrogen to feed the bacteria. Make sure each layer is moist but not drenched. Finally, cover the bin with old carpet or some similar lid to keep in the heat.

You will need to turn the compost out into the second bin to achieve the best results. When you do this depends on the time of year, after three or four weeks in summer or after about four months in winter. The process adds air and aids decomposition.

The compost should heat up when first made to at least 60°C (140°F). This is essential for killing weed seeds. The compost is ready to use when it has become dark and crumbly.

Avoid putting leaves in your heap because they take longer to decompose. You need a separate bin for leaves; one made of wire will be sufficient. The leaves will rot down in two years, sometimes longer with plane leaves, less with oak and beech. If you have a shredder it will reduce this time to one year, or alternatively you can run a rotary mower over leaves dropped onto lawn areas to chop them up before composting.

When you see the prices of delivered organic compost you will be glad you made your own, as well as having solved the problem of how to deal with your household and garden waste.

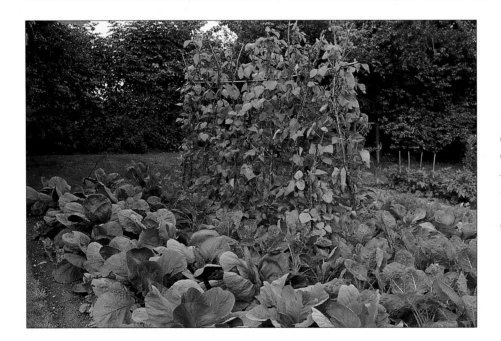

Vegetable plots can be highly ornamental, not only with the flowers of crops but also with varied foliage colour. Members of the brassica family usually have glaucous leaves, tinged with reddish purple in the case of the 'red cabbage' here.

shrivel them in no time and repay all your effort. Hoeing in wet weather is a fool's game, as many will re-root. Suppress weeds in the ornamental garden by densely planting groundcover species. If necessary hand weed until the groundcover is fully established.

Coping with pests and diseases

Pests and diseases can often be prevented at an early stage by good hygiene and other cultural controls such as selecting varieties that have been bred for their resistance to pest and disease. If you do get a problem, there are several solutions that avoid the type of chemicals that may persist in the environment and damage wildlife. One of the best remedies in the greenhouse is to use predators of the pest or disease. First you will need to identify the particular problem, and there are several handbooks that will help (see Further Reading on page 156).

You can acquire the predator from an amateur supplier, who will generally give advice about when to introduce it, the optimum temperature for it to establish and when further introductions are needed. (A List of Suppliers is given on page 157.) This 'biological control' is a question of balance, so you can never hope to eliminate the problem totally; organic gardening inevitably means accepting some level of pest damage. The main biological controls available are: *Encarsia formosa* for glasshouse whitefly, *Phytoseuilus persimilis* for red spider mite, *Aphidoletes* or *Verticillium lecani* for aphids, *Cryptoleimus monstrosus* for mealy bug and *Bacillus thuringiensis* for various caterpillars.

There are some sprays you can use if absolutely necessary. Soft soap causes pests to fall off the plants. Other sprays such as pyrethum or derris that are recommended as 'organic' may not be toxic to many parts of the food chain but can be harmful to fish and other aquatic life. So avoid using them on plants near pools.

A further alternative is to deter pests by 'companion planting', using plants that excrete deterrent chemicals. For example, onions planted densely near carrots deter carrot root fly and French beans near cabbages deter cabbage root fly.

Other physical deterrents include putting greasebands around fruit trees in the autumn to prevent pests ascending to overwinter in the bark, and paper collars on brassicas to prevent the cabbage root fly laying her eggs.

Hand-picking is a last resort used, for example, to reduce slugs and snails. One of my abiding memories of visiting a smallholding in Maine, USA, was joining the Colorado beetle 'detail' every day, picking the plump larvae off the potato leaves and summoning up the nerve to squash kilos of them underfoot. If you can do this you have really come of age as an organic gardener!

This garden at the Chelsea Flower Show makes plentiful use of colourful tagetes among the asparagus and red cabbage. The terracottas are rhubarb-forcing pots.

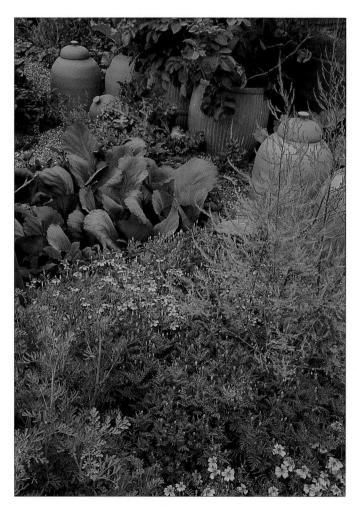

GROWING HEALTHY VEGETABLES

○

If you have a small garden you may well choose to grow a proportion of the vegetables you eat. You can enjoy the benefit of extra-fresh supplies picked a few minutes before going into the pot by sowing little and often. If you have an allotment or large vegetable plot you are likely to produce enough crops to store over winter or to freeze. Allotments can take up a lot of time, especially if you are inheriting a weed-ridden patch. The vegetables you produce will not work out cheaper if you cost the time of your own labour, so be sure your effort will give you enjoyment. It will certainly help your fitness!

The great advantages of growing your own vegetables include not only the speed with which you can get them from garden to table but also

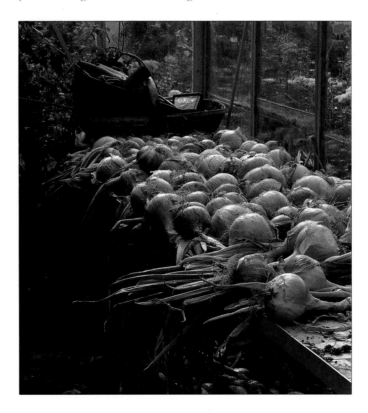

Onions are easily grown from sets (small bulbs). They need to dry off thoroughly to store well through the winter.

the unusual types you can choose to grow. Such produce may not be easily available in the shops. You can also choose to grow organically and know that your produce contains no residues. No one knows if these residues are harmful in accumulation, in combination with one another, and over time, so avoiding them is probably wise.

Choosing what to grow

First of all, do not attempt to grow vegetables in the heart of urban areas or near busy roads. The fallout of lead from traffic fumes can be significant, especially on to leafy vegetables. If you have a small garden I would recommend growing all your salad requirements – lettuce, salad onions, radish, spinach, beetroot and so on. Sow little and often to avoid a glut. Coriander is particularly tasty in green salads but runs to seed quickly, like radish, so sow a little every ten days.

Decide what are your favourite vegetables and what you have room for. The commercial production of peas is so good now that you may decide that your space is better used to grow mangetout peas, which anyway are rather expensive in the shops. If you particularly like young turnips, grow these, especially if you can grow them fast with a lot of water. Turnips are difficult to buy as they are usually grown to maturity to feed cattle. Root crops such as parsnips, carrots and potatoes take up a lot of ground, so you may decide these are not for you. Onions grown from sets, and leeks, however, are very productive from a small piece of ground. If you like marrows and squashes, grow the bush varieties rather than the trailers as they are more compact. Make full use of cloches to grow winter hardy lettuce varieties and cauliflowers to mature in the spring – these are normally sprayed repeatedly with fungicides by commercial growers.

If you have an allotment or a large vegetable garden you will almost certainly want to grow potatoes. You can choose from a range of varieties

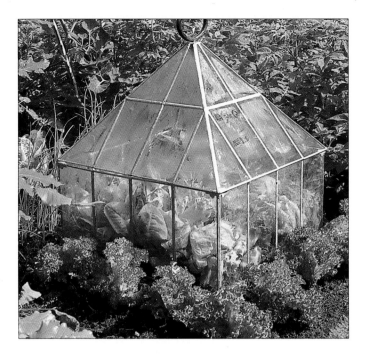

Extend your growing season and cover tender crops by using Victorian lantern cloches now available as replicas, at a price!

to buy as sets to plant in mid spring and you can choose ones that are either unavailable in the shops or very expensive. Excellent salad varieties include 'Belle de Fontenay' and 'Pink Fir Apple'. The latter is also a particularly good keeper; it can be lifted or harvested in late autumn and stored until the following spring. Commercial varieties of maincrop potatoes are sprayed with maleic hydrazide after harvesting to inhibit them sprouting in store. Tests by the National Vegetable Station in Britain have shown that pesticides, like vitamins and minerals, are concentrated just under the skin of most vegetables. So by growing your own potatoes you can eat the skins (and get the benefit of the fibre) with peace of mind. The same applies to carrots, which are best peeled to rid residues of pesticides sprayed for carrot root fly, unless you have grown your own.

Certain vegetables are grown commercially with very little pesticide simply because breeders have developed good disease-resistant varieties. From the point of view of avoiding residues, therefore, you may not wish to bother growing parsnips, or beetroots for winter storing; or even onions or leeks, though they may have been treated with a fungicide. Lettuce sold in mid summer has often been grown very fast without artificial fertilizers or pesticides and so is virtually organic. A healthy aphid on such a lettuce is probably a good sign!

Do not exhaust the soil in your vegetable garden by continuous cropping. Rotate your crops according to the pattern shown in the box. If you practise good rotation and soil management you should produce excellent crops organically.

ROTATING YOUR CROPS

Divide the plot into four.

Plant potatoes in one section, peas and beans in the second, root vegetables in the third, and cucurbits and brassicas in the fourth. Rotate the cycle each year.

Dig in manure before you plant cucurbits and brassicas. This will be used up by the following year and will not overfeed the root vegetables, which causes them to fork. The peas and beans make their own feed in their roots by taking nitrogen from the air, so need no fertilizers. If you leave their roots in after cropping they will help to feed the succeeding potatoes, although you can augment this by using fish, blood and bone fertilizer, an excellent organic substitute for the all-purpose chemical fertilizers. The manure is far enough away from the potatoes in the rotation to prevent scab disease.

In this way the vegetable garden feeds itself and the soil is well looked after.

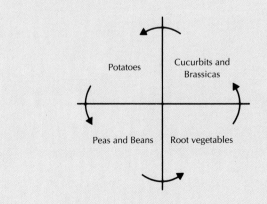

FRESH FRUIT

○

Fruit is an important part of a healthy balanced diet; it helps supply vitamins, minerals and plenty of fibre to assist the digestive system. If you have a fairly large garden you can grow a wide variety of fruit yourself, with the advantage of knowing that your produce is free of the pesticides that commercial fruit farmers use.

Growing your own soft fruit

Soft fruit can be considered in three categories. Cane fruit, such as raspberries, blackberries, tayberries and loganberries, produce fruit on canes that need to be supported. Bush fruits, such as black, red and white currants, blueberries and gooseberries, grow on free-standing bushes. The third category is fruit produced on ground-hugging plants; wild and cultivated strawberries are the best examples.

If you have a professional attitude to gardening you will grow all your soft fruit in a cotton or nylon mesh fruit cage to prevent bird damage. It is always worth investing in a treated timber post and wire support for your cane fruit.

Buy dormant one or two-year-old canes and

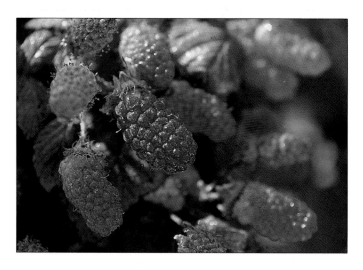

Tayberries produce a luscious, relatively acid-free fruit, less tart than loganberries, and they freeze well.

plant them in well-manured soil some time in the winter when the ground is not frozen. Plant raspberries 45cm (18in) apart and the other soft fruits 2.4 metres (8ft) apart to allow for training the canes. Most raspberries fruit on the previous year's canes, so prune out canes that have fruited and tie in the new growth. (Exceptions are the delicious autumn-fruiting varieties such as 'Autumn Bliss' which fruit on current growth and are pruned in early winter.) Blackberries, tayberries and loganberries are pruned after fruiting; take out the old growth and tie in the new. All cane fruits are excellent for freezing.

Plant bush fruits 1.5 metres (5ft) apart as two-year-old bushes. Again, prepare the ground well and plant during mild weather in the dormant season. Prune bush fruit during winter. Aim to take out a third of the old wood of black currants. Red and white currants and gooseberries are spur pruned; that is, their side growth is cut back to within 7cm (2½in) of the stems. They then produce fruit on these spurs.

Blueberries should be planted as dormant plants into acid ground, 1.2 metres (4ft) apart, or you can try growing them in the ornamental garden among other shrubs. They fruit in late summer. Cut out a proportion of the oldest shoots in winter to keep up the vigour of the plant.

Strawberries are best planted as young pot-grown runners in late summer so that they can become established before winter. Set them 30cm (12in) apart into well-manured soil. The plants will crop well for three years, providing you remove the runners. Replace the stock after this time. Strawberries need 'strawing up' in early summer; this involves placing straw under the leaves and young fruit to keep them clean for picking. You can put cloches over strawberries to obtain early crops, or grow them in strawberry pots on the patio. Strawberries grown in these pots are quite successful if you do not allow the soil to dry out.

Growing your own tree fruit

You can grow quite a variety of tree or 'top' fruit in a relatively small space, providing you pay attention to training methods and getting the right rootstock.

One of the problems with tree fruit as opposed to soft fruit is pollination, particularly with apples, pears, cherries and, to a lesser extent, plums. In a small garden where you cannot plant two varieties to ensure pollination, plant a 'family' tree; that is, one that has a number of varieties grafted on to it.

Apples and pears can be grown as free-standing trees on a rootstock chosen to produce the size of tree suitable for your garden. Alternatively they can be trained against a wall or against a post and wire fence. Cordon trees produce fruit on spurs off a single stem trained at forty-five degrees. Espalier trees fruit on spurs produced on tiers of horizontal branches. Low espaliers (with one or two tiers) make attractive divisions in the fruit garden or can be used in place of hedges.

Plums, gages and cherries can often be bought as fan-trained trees, ready to plant against a wall. The sour Morello cherry (delicious in pies) is an excellent choice for a shady wall. Apricots, peaches and nectarines are also available as fans but may be expensive. They must be planted against a very warm wall and need no pollinator varieties, but you must be prepared to train in the shoots. Imagine presenting your own fruit at a party!

This espaliered apple has been trained on into an arch.

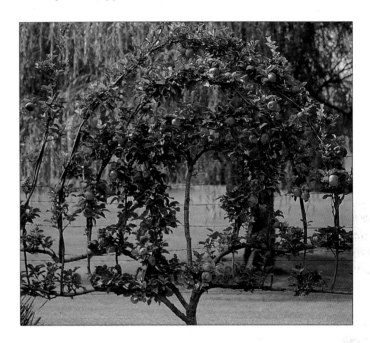

RECOMMENDED VARIETIES

Soft fruit		Top fruit	
Blackberries	Bedford Giant	Apples	James Grieve with Queen Cox
	Oregon Thornless (for the patio)		or Ribston Pippin with Egremont
Black currants	Baldwin		Russet
	Ben Lomond	Apricots	Moorpark
Blueberries	Bluecrop		Farmingdale
	Herbert	Cherries	Stella (self-fertile)
Gooseberries	White Smith		or Van with Merton Glory
	Whinham's Industry	Gages	Oullins Golden Gage (self-fertile)
Loganberries	Thornless		Old Greengage (self-fertile)
	LY 59 (a virus-free type)	Nectarines	Elruge
Raspberries	Malling Jewel		Lord Napier
	Autumn Bliss	Peaches	Rochester
Red currants	Red Lake	Pears	Doyenne du Comice with
Strawberries	Royal Sovereign (if you can		Winter Nellis
	obtain it virus free)	Plums	Coe's Golden Drop with
White currants	White Versailles		Dennison's Superb

A WIDER RANGE OF FRUIT AND VEGETABLES

Growing something out of the ordinary can give you a real sense of achievement besides yielding ingredients for more adventurous meals. There is a range of fruits and vegetables that are simply uncommon, not necessarily because they are difficult to grow, though some of them need the shelter of a warm wall.

Unusual fruits

Actinidia deliciosa Chinese Gooseberry or Kiwi Fruit.
This delicious green fruit is healthily low in calories and extremely high in vitamin C, and is excellent as a dessert fruit, in fruit salads and pavlovas. The female vines on which it grows need pollinating by a male plant. Grow in full sun.

Cydonia oblonga Quince
The quince is a small tree which produces quite large pale pink flowers in late spring and pear-like fruit that ripen in mid autumn. They make an excellent jam or jelly, can be candied with sugar or used to make 'quince cheese', a delicious dessert dish.

Cyphomandra crassicaulis Tamarillo
This is sometimes called the Tree Tomato because it produces fruits rather like an oval plum tomato, though they are sharper in taste. In Britain the plant needs cultivation under glass. Its fruits are good in tarts and are high in vitamin C.

Diospyros kaki Persimmon or Sharon Fruit
This fruit is native to China and Japan and will only bear fruit in a warm climate such as the Mediterranean area, Australia or the southern USA. It is a tall tree and produces orange, astringent fruits reminiscent of a tomato. They are delicious candied.

Eriobotrya japonica Loquat
This is an elegant small tree or large shrub that needs a sheltered sunny spot to produce its yellow fruits that appear in the spring, following an autumn flowering. Native to China and Japan, it is widely planted throughout the Mediterranean region. Eat loquats in pies; they are a good source of vitamins.

Ficus carica Fig
Figs need a very warm and sheltered spot, preferably on a sunny wall. Constrict their roots in a brick-built box 60cm (2½ft) square by as much deep, sunken into the ground at the foot of the wall. This will encourage fruit at the expense of leaf growth. The variety 'Brown Turkey' is a classic. Figs are a gentle laxative.

Mespilus germanica Medlar
The medlar is a small tree that flowers in early summer and is a member of the rose family. Its curious brown fruits never ripen fully in Britain but are picked in late autumn and allowed to become *almost* rotten before eating. This 'bletted' fruit is then enjoyed as a delicacy with port or madeira. It has a granular texture and, to my mind, tastes like a rich pear. Plant a named variety, such as 'Nottingham' or 'Dutch' in a sunny position in a well-drained soil.

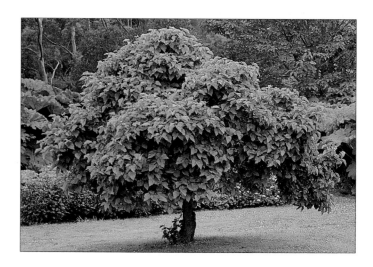

Mulberries produce a spreading shape and are very long lived.

Morus nigra Mulberry
Mulberries are almost never available commercially; the fruit must be fully ripe when picked and will not stand market handling. A mulberry tree will produce fruit when quite young and trees live to a great age. A tip when the tree is of a good size is to naturalize bulbs under it and not mow under it until mid summer. This means that when the fruit matures in late summer and some inevitably drops it will not mark a prized lawn! Mulberries make excellent jam and wine, and are delicious with ice cream.

Physalis peruviana Cape Gooseberry
Once cultivated around the Cape of Good Hope, this perennial plant produces a slightly acid, bright yellow berry with an inflated calyx. The berries make curious novelties as dessert fruits, and are easy to grow in any soil in slight shade.

Punica granatum Pomegranate
This Asian fruit is now naturalized throughout the subtropics. It can be grown in England on a very warm wall for interest, although the best fruits are grown in the Mediterranean. They have an acid, seedy pulp rather like a passion fruit, and are quite a good laxative. A pomegranate tree fruits regularly at the Chelsea Physic Garden adjacent to the bell once rung by student apothecaries to gain admission.

Unusual vegetables

Abelmoschus esculentus Okra
This is quite easy to crop from seed in warm gardens and it produces very beautiful, though ephemeral, flowers before setting the large pods sometimes known as 'Ladies Fingers'. This rather mucilaginous vegetable is popular in curries, and it has a high ratio of fibre to flesh. Indians know Okra as 'bhindi'.

Apium graveolens var. rapaceum Celeriac or Turnip-rooted Celery
This is a useful vegetable to grow if you have heavy soil in which celery will not grow well. Grate the swollen root and eat it in salads dressed with lemon juice. It is a good source of fibre.

Asparagus officinalis Asparagus
This is an excellent crop to grow to save money because asparagus is always expensive to buy. However, you need soil that is free of perennial weeds, quite a bit of space to lay out a bed, patience (it takes several years to crop from two-year-old roots) and discipline (it should not be picked after mid summer or you will run down the strength of the plants). If you can manage all this, enjoy it with butter as a delicious source of fibre.

Brassicas Rare and various
Besides the usual sprouts and cabbages there is a range of unusual varieties much grown by the

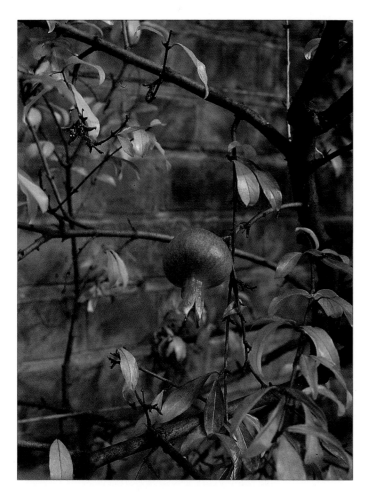

A pomegranate in autumn light at the Chelsea Physic Garden.

HOW TO GROW TROPICAL FRUIT PLANTS FROM PIPS

Many attractive plants can be grown easily from the pips of tropical fruits. All you need is a simple electric propagator to provide a good temperature, a good compost and enough light when the seeds have germinated. This is a hobby that adults and children alike find fascinating. How delightful to have your own miniature fruit orchard! Here are some suggestions of fruits easily available in supermarkets.

Fruit	Botanical name	Germination method	Temperature	Compost
Avocado	*Persea americana*	Part submerge in water with the pointed end uppermost. Pot on when shoot/root is well emerged.	18°C (65°F) (ambient room temperature)	
Cherimoya	*Annona cherimola*	Plant in compost, with the seed just covered.	21°C (70°F)	John Innes No.2
Christophine	*Sechium edule*	Plant the large single seed part-covered by compost.	16°C (60°F)	John Innes No.2
Date*	*Phoenix dactylifera*	Place in moist vermiculite in a polythene bag in a propagator or airing cupboard. Pot each one up once a root has emerged.	21°C (70°F)	John Innes No.1
Grapefruit	*Citrus × paradisi*	Sow fresh seeds from really ripe fruit. Plant shallowly.	16–21°C (60–70°F)	John Innes Seed Compost
Guava	*Psidium guajava*	Sow fresh seed.	16–21°C (60–70°F)	John Innes Seed Compost
Kumquat	*Fortunella* sp.	As for grapefruit.	16°C (60°F)	John Innes Seed Compost
Loquat	*Eriobotrya japonica*	As for grapefruit.	13°C (55°F)	John Innes Seed Compost
Mango*	*Mangifera indica*	Plant the flattened stone sharp edge down.	21–24°C (70–75°F)	John Innes No.2
Passion fruit	*Passiflora edulis*	Sow fresh seed in its pulp.	18°C (65°F)	John Innes No.2
Pawpaw	*Carica papaya*	Sow fresh seed.	18°C (65°F)	John Innes No.2
Pomegranate	*Punica granatum*	Sow fresh or dried seed in spring.	21°C (70°F)	John Innes Seed Compost
Rambutan	*Nephelium lappaceum*	Sow fresh seed.	21–24°C (70–75°F)	John Innes Seed Compost
Starfruit	*Averrhoa carambola*	Sow fresh seed.	21°C (70°F)	John Innes Seed Compost

*Cover seed with very hot (*not* boiling) water and leave to soak for twenty-four hours before sowing.

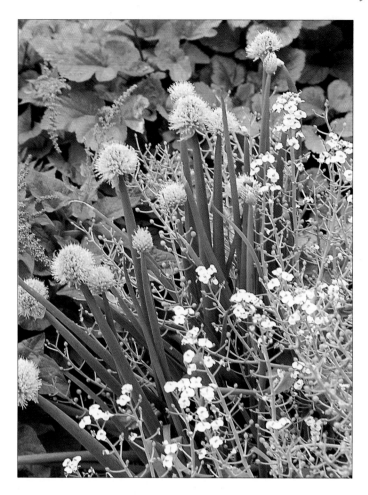

Seakale (bottom right); pretty in flower and tasty to eat, and grown here with Welsh onions.

Crambe maritima Seakale
This is an attractive seaside plant with grey-green leaves and white flowers. If you lift roots in the autumn, pot them up and put them in the dark in an airing cupboard or warm cellar you can force the young shoots. These have a nutty flavour and are a welcome salad vegetable for the winter when there is a shortage of vitamin-rich fresh produce.

Cynara scolymus Globe Artichoke
This is a handsome thistle-like plant with a blue flower, worthy of a place in the flower border. As a bonus you can cut the unopened flowerhead and boil it, using the fleshy base of each petal dipped in butter as an appetizer. I always feel the time involved in dismantling the flower is an appetizer in itself! This plant is not to be confused with *Helianthus tuberosus* Jerusalem Artichoke, which produces nutty-flavoured tubers in great profusion. These are an excellent source of fibre and contain a sweetener that can be digested by diabetics. In a good summer the plants will produce flowers like small sunflowers, but beware, each plant is enormously productive. So do not plant too many or you will have an embarrassment of riches!

Scorzonera hispanica Scorzonera
This is a black-skinned root vegetable with a sweet white flesh digestible by diabetics. If you leave it in the ground for a second season its roots are larger and easier to crop.

Solanum melongena Aubergine
This is a crop really worth growing under glass in Britain rather like Sweet Peppers, and just as easy to grow, providing you introduce a predator against whitefly. Use it in ratatouille or as a fruit that can be stuffed with a meat or vegetable filling. It is also an essential ingredient of Greek moussaka. Do not eat aubergines raw.

Tragopon porrifolius Salsify
This root vegetable is grown in the same way as scorzonera but tastes rather like oysters. It is sometimes known as the Vegetable Oyster. Salsify is very good in a creamed soup.

Chinese and used in stir fries. The secret of these Chinese Greens is to grow them quickly in a moist soil with a lot of water and eat them young. Kohlrabi is a useful variety, sometimes known as Turnip-rooted Cabbage. Grow this in the same way and you can enjoy its nutty flavour when lightly boiled to preserve the vitamins.

Capsicum annuum Sweet Pepper
I remember growing these in 1973 when they were a novel crop in Britain. They are more common now, but really require cultivation in a cold greenhouse or under tall cloches where they are no more difficult than tomatoes. They are delicious raw or cooked.

GARLIC: THE 'HEAL ALL'

Garlic is the one member of the onion family that has extensive use in medicine as well as in cooking. Thought originally to come from Asia, it has a long history of use throughout the world. The Egyptians gave an allowance of garlic to their slaves to keep up their strength, Greek athletes considered that it gave them energy, and the Romans valued it greatly.

Medicinal uses of garlic

The Greek physician Galen called garlic the 'heal all' and throughout history it has been used for a variety of problems – as an antibiotic and an expectorant, and to treat thrombosis, worms, leprosy and even diabetes. Culpeper recommended garlic to heal skin diseases and believed that there were few problems that it would not help. The Chinese use it to treat digestive problems, whooping cough and skin diseases, and it has been shown in trials to reduce blood cholesterol levels.

In medieval times garlic was used as an ingredient of 'thieves vinegar' with which thieves would protect themselves while robbing the bodies of plague victims. Garlic is commonly used in herbal medicine and was helpful as an emergency antiseptic in World War One. The antibiotic effects of garlic are thought to be due to allicin, named from its botanical name *Allium sativum*, and which is the constituent of the essential oils of garlic that give its characteristic smell.

With such a repertoire of uses, it is not surprising that garlic has entered folklore. Throughout the Middle and Far East, garlic cloves have been carried to protect against evil (hence the origin of its common name 'Devil's Posy') and from medieval times it was thought to be both an aphrodisiac and able to repel vampires.

Garlic in cooking

In Britain garlic was eschewed as 'peasant's food' in the Middle Ages and was known pejoratively as 'camphor of the poor'. The French and Italians,

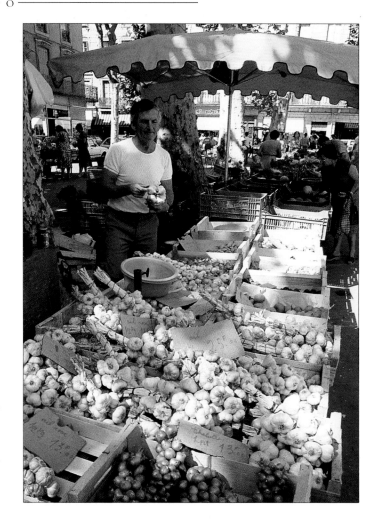

Ropes of garlic bulbs for sale in the market of the town of Carcassonne, Languedoc, southern France.

however, have always enjoyed using garlic in their cuisines, and the French hold special feasts at the time of the garlic harvest, with every item on the menu containing it. Aïoli (garlic mayonnaise) is a particular favourite in France. In Gilroy, California, which supplies the USA with its garlic, there is an annual festival that is celebrated with great razzmatazz.

The pervasive smell of garlic is released from the various sulphurous compounds it contains when the tissues are crushed. These odours can be absorbed by the intestine or by the skin and then exhaled or emitted from the skin. People who find garlic unpleasant can take it medicinally in capsules that are tasteless, or take soup where the boiling has removed the smell. Parsley is known to reduce its smell on the breath.

The main producers of garlic are now Spain, Egypt and Argentina, though it is also a significant crop in China, Thailand, France and Italy. On a world scale, garlic is the second most important allium crop after *Allium cepa*, the onion. The best areas for cultivation in Britain are the warm areas of the south coast and Isle of Wight. For people who enjoy collecting wild food and prefer mild garlic, it is a good idea to collect Ramsons *Allium ursinum*, a pretty woodland species with broad leaves and white flowerheads. Collect this in areas which are too cool and damp to grow well-flavoured true garlic.

21-BULB GARLIC SOUP

For a dinner party of at least eight and said to be very curative after too much alcohol.

21 BULBS (not cloves) of garlic
2.4 litres (4 pts) of water
Bouquet garni
Salt and pepper
4 tablespoons olive oil
75g (3 oz) butter
50g (2 oz) flour
2 eggs

Separate the cloves and drop them into boiling water for one minute. Then strain and peel them (allow enough time!). Put them into the water, add the bouquet garni, salt and pepper to taste and the oil, and bring to the boil.

Allow the soup to simmer for an hour and crush any remaining cloves into a pulp with a wooden spoon. Melt the butter and add the flour to it, then stir the mixture into the soup.

Allow the soup to cool slightly and then stir in two well-beaten eggs. Serve with fresh bread.

HOW TO GROW GARLIC

Obtain large, firm garlic bulbs and divide them into individual cloves. Reject the small ones (use them for cooking) and plant the largest cloves 3–4cm (1½in) deep and 15cm (6in) apart in well-manured ground in full sun. Plant in late autumn, or early spring in areas with cold, wet winters. Keep the bed free of weeds and remove the flowerheads when they appear. Allow the crop to die down in mid summer and harvest the bulbs in late summer. Dry them off on a rack in a cool, dry, well-ventilated shed. Store them in strings (like onions), or loose in a netted bag in an airy room with a temperature under 20°C (68°F).

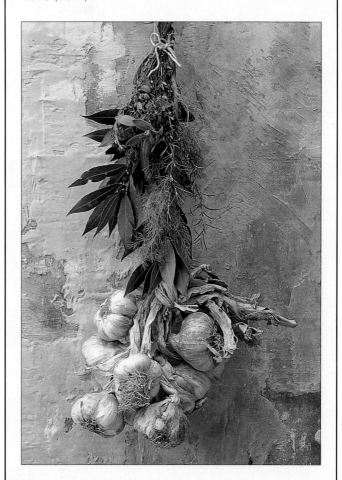

Garlic is best stored in a cool, well-ventilated outhouse. Combine it with herbs to make a superb soup.

MEDICINAL HERBS

T here are a number of herbs which are useful as remedies for minor ailments and have been used as such over many years. The table opposite describes how to grow and use the plant medicinally. The glossary below summarizes the main methods of treatment used in folk medi-cine, in 'over the counter' preparations (sold without a doctor's prescription) and as dispensed by medical herbalists. Only self-treat minor problems and seek help if an ailment persists, because you might be confusing an apparently minor problem with a more deep-seated illness.

A GLOSSARY OF TREATMENT METHODS

Compress	Lint or cotton wool dipped into a herbal infusion (see below) and applied externally. Compresses can be applied hot or (more commonly) cold to reduce bruising etc. External herbal treatment by compress was common in many traditions of ethnic medicine (see also Poultice).
Decoction	The liquid produced when a herb is boiled and imparts its healing properties to the liquid.
Infusion	The liquid produced when a herb has been covered with boiling water for several minutes. This is the commonest method of producing a herbal tea, but some are made by decoction (see above).
Oil	The mixture produced when a herb has infused its potency into vegetable oil and a small amount of vinegar over a period of weeks and in a warm place. These oils can be used in therapeutic massage.
Ointment	A paste for external application produced by adding crushed herbs to melted petroleum jelly and simmering for about twenty minutes.
Poultice	A soft, hot mixture of fresh herbs briefly boiled in muslin and applied externally. Poultices are common practice in many traditions of ethnic medicine.
Syrup	The result of adding sugar to a herbal infusion and simmering until the consistency is syrupy. Often used for minor ailments in children as a more palatable medicine.
Tincture	A herbal extract preserved in alcohol in which it will keep indefinitely. Tinctures are the commonest method of prescription by medical herbalists.

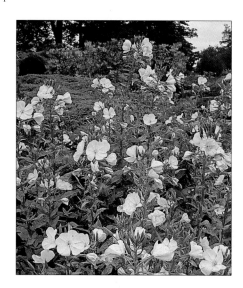

Evening primrose heals eczema.

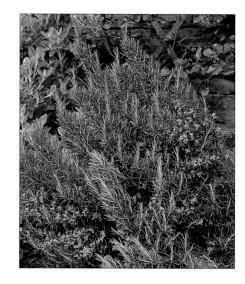

Rosemary oil is used in embrocation.

PLANT REMEDIES FOR MINOR ILLS

Common name/Botanical name	Cultivation	Application/Medicinal use
Aloe *Aloe vera*	As a pot plant in a sunny window.	As an ointment for minor muscular aches.
Anise *Pimpinella anisum*	Sow seed in late spring.	A hot infusion for indigestion.
Arnica *Arnica montana*	Sow seed in late spring.	As an ointment for bruising.
Caraway *Carum carvi*	Sow seed in late spring.	Chew the seeds for indigestion or flatulence.
Comfrey *Symphytum officinale*	Sow seed in early spring.	Crushed leaves as a cold compress for bruising.
Coriander *Coriandrum sativum*	Sow seed in late spring.	A hot infusion for indigestion.
Elderflower *Sambucus nigra*	Sow seed in late summer.	A hot infusion for slight fever.
Evening Primrose *Oenothera biennis*	Sow seed in late spring.	An external application as an oil for eczema.
Eyebright *Euphrasia officinalis*	Seed (you may need to collect small quantities from pastureland).	A hot infusion for hayfever.
Hypericum *Hypericum perforatum*	Sow seed in early spring.	Massage with the oil for bruising – or apply to cuts.
Hyssop *Hyssopus officinalis*	Sow seed in early spring.	A hot infusion for slight fever.
Lemon Balm *Melissa officinalis*	Sow seed in early spring.	A hot infusion for headache.
Lime Blossom *Tilia × vulgaris*	Collect from mature trees.	A hot infusion for headache.
Marjoram *Origanum marjorana* and *O. vulgare*	Sow in late spring.	Apply as an oil for minor muscular aches or on lint to an aching tooth.
Nasturtium *Tropaeolum majus*	Sow in late spring.	Crush the seeds and make a poultice to apply to styes.
Parsley *Petroselinum crispum*	Sow in late spring.	Make a cold compress of crushed leaves to apply to insect bites.
Peppermint *Mentha × piperita*	Sow in early spring.	A hot infusion for indigestion.
Rosemary *Rosmarinus officinalis*	Take cuttings in early spring. Needs a warm spot to thrive.	Apply as an oil for minor muscular aches.
Thyme *Thymus vulgaris*	Sow in early spring.	Make a tincture and gargle with it to alleviate a sore throat.
Valerian *Valeriana officinalis*	Sow seed in early spring.	Make a cold decoction of the root to alleviate nervous tension.
Witch Hazel *Hamamelis virginiana*	Obtain a young plant (it is very slow from seed).	Make a cold compress of the bark to alleviate bruising or make an ointment to apply to small wounds.
Yarrow *Achillea millefolium*	Sow seed in early spring.	Apply as an ointment to chilblains.

HERBAL TEAS TO REFRESH AND HEAL

O ne of the commonest ways in which you can enjoy the gentle healing properties of herbs is by drinking infusions or herbal teas. The flavour of herbal teas makes a welcome alternative to the caffeine-based beverages of tea and coffee, and can be enjoyed hot in winter or cooled and iced in summer. There are several proprietary brands of herb teas available in sachet form but it is much more fun (and considerably cheaper) to use herbs from your own garden.

You should allow about three teaspoons of the fresh herb per cup of boiling water and the tea will be much more flavourful if you crush the leaves beforehand. In winter you can make use of dried herbs, but these must be kept in opaque glass airtight jars or tins to retain their flavour, much like ordinary teas. Allow the tea to steep for about five minutes before straining and drinking. Add honey to taste if required.

CULPEPER'S ADVICE

Camomile Flower

'easeth ... all pains and torments of the belly.'

Lemon Balm

'driveth away all troublesome care and thoughts out of the mind, arising from melancholy and black choler.'

Peppermint

'This herb has a strong, agreeable, aromatic smell ... it is useful for complaints of the stomach, such as wind, vomiting, etc., for which there are few remedies of greater efficacy.'

Thyme

'The herb taken inwardly, comforts the stomach much, and expels wind.'

ABOVE RIGHT: Nicholas Culpeper, the seventeenth-century herbalist, wrote his advice in English rather than Latin so that his recommendations could be followed more easily by the 'common people'.

RIGHT: Bergamot Monarda didyma is known in the USA as Oswego Tea. The flowers can be simmered to make an oily herbal tea. Bergamot is not the species used to scent Earl Grey tea; that perfume is conveyed by spraying the tea with the oil of Citrus bergamia, the so-called 'Bergamot orange' of Calabria.

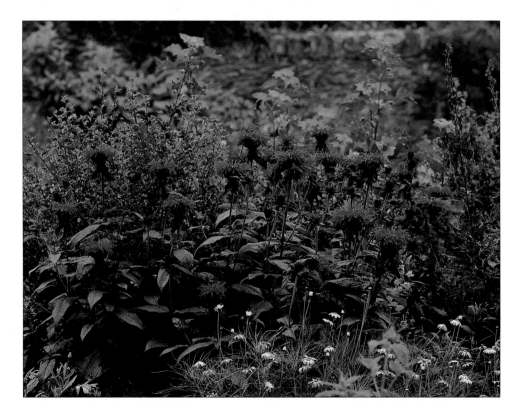

A TABLE OF HERBAL TEAS

Herb	Botanical name	Therapeutic effect	Special notes
Bergamot Flower	*Monarda didyma*	Induces sleep.	Simmer the tea rather than infuse.
Camomile Flower	*Chamaemelum nobile*	Induces sleep. Good for head colds, headaches and stomach aches.	Steep for only a few minutes to produce a mild brew.
Hop Flower	*Humulus lupulus*	Induces sleep.	Steep for only a few minutes to produce a mild brew.
Horsetail	*Equisetum* spp.	Calms an upset stomach.	Soak the dried herb for an hour. Boil and then simmer for ten minutes. Strain after ten minutes and drink.
Lemon Balm	*Melissa officinalis*	Relaxing. Reduces restlessness. Induces sweating in colds/influenza. Seek medical help if fever persists.	Useful bedtime drink.
Lemon Verbena	*Aloysia triphylla*	Induces sleep.	Infuse for two minutes only as this is very strongly flavoured.
Lime (Linden) Blossom	*Tilia × vulgaris*	Relaxing, induces sleep. Improves blood circulation.	Do not steep for more than a few minutes.
Peppermint	*Mentha × piperita*	Relieves indigestion, flatulence, colic, nausea, fever, morning sickness in pregnancy. An excellent all-round digestive.	Do not use if taking homoeopathic remedies as peppermint is said to antidote them, especially when taken internally.
Rose Hip	*Rosa canina*	Tonic.	Use dried hips and infuse for seven minutes. Rose hips are a valuable source of vitamin C.
Sage	*Salvia officinalis*	Stress.	Best not used in pregnancy.
Thyme	*Thymus vulgaris* or *T. × citriodorus*	Reduces headaches. Acts as a general tonic to the whole system.	Infuse for ten minutes.
Valerian Root	*Valeriana officinalis*	Very effective for stress and anxiety.	Infuse in cold water for twenty-four hours. Cold infusions take far longer than hot ones.
Verbascum	*Verbascum thapsus*	Reduces coughs.	Infuse for ten minutes and strain through muslin.
Woodruff	*Galium odoratum*	Invigorating, refreshing.	Infuse for an hour in hot water. Drink cold with lemon and honey.

DESIGNING A HERB GARDEN

○

Growing and using herbs is becoming increasingly popular. These attractive aromatic plants take little space so that even urban gardeners can find ways of having their own small herb garden, whether simply a herb pot on the windowsill, a window box or a small border close to the house. Planning and planting a special area for herbs in the garden can add an unusual and useful feature, providing a link to one of gardening's oldest traditions.

The herb garden tradition

The strongest tradition in the design of herb gardens is that of the formal monastery courtyard. In the Middle Ages herbs for medicinal or culinary use were grown close to the monastery's hospital and kitchens, just as they had been in the early gardens of Roman Pompeii. A modern construction can be seen in the Kitchen Court of Emmanuel College, Cambridge, designed in 1961.

These gardens were always formal, with the beds edged in some way, either with low hedges or reed fencing, so that the herbs could be gathered easily. The formality of the design reflected the order of the monks' highly structured lives. Most of the gardens were quartered in design, with some focal point in the centre, and this then became a tradition in many sixteenth and seventeenth-century physic gardens. This layout can still be seen at the Chelsea Physic Garden today, though the herb garden and medicinal plants are confined to one quadrant.

Planning your own design

An advantage of creating a formal design is that it allows you to control the rather lax shape of growth of many herbs that look pleasing in spring but can become formless and tired by the end of

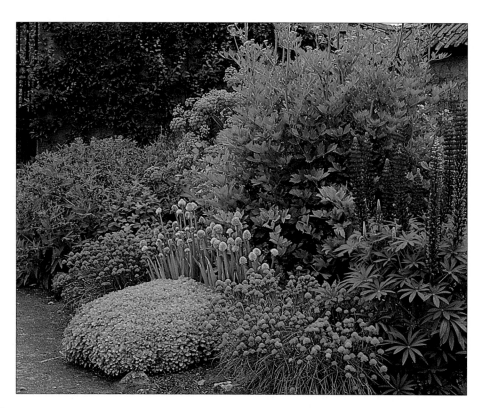

ABOVE RIGHT: *Small formal herb gardens are often designed as a 'herb wheel' centred by a feature. Here, the path surfaces help reflect the sun's warmth to the benefit of the low creeping thymes, but would need to be far wider to allow access for wheelchair users.*

LEFT: *Many herbs are ornamental enough in flower to be successfully accommodated in a mixed border such as that at Barrington Court in Somerset, England. The foliage and flowers of lovage, angelica, southernwood, comfrey, golden marjoram, balm and chives tone happily with the lupin.*

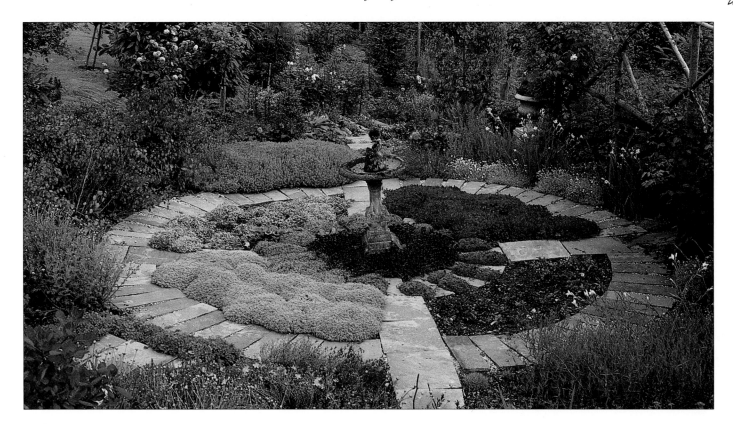

summer. Neatly clipped hedges and straight paths can counter the formless effect and topiary can give vertical accent.

The divisions of the garden can be useful in differentiating the herbs by their uses. A 'herb wheel', where each segment is planted with a variety separated from its neighbour by a 'spoke' of brick or stone, is a design that can be adapted easily to any size of garden. There is a good recent example at Stockeld Park in Wetherby, North Yorkshire, England.

· In the traditional designs of herb gardens the beds are often surrounded by walls, perhaps the better to contain the aromatic volatile oils of many species. Some of these plants only release their oils when crushed, so a delightful way of enjoying them is to grow them in raised beds where they are easily touched, a particular pleasure for the partially sighted or wheelchair users. Well-placed seats, planted with a low bed of camomile, and perhaps arbours, make attractive havens for enjoying the perfumes in peace.

HOW TO MARK OUT A 'HERB WHEEL'

Choose the maximum diameter you desire in an area of full sun unobstructed by overhanging trees. Choose your centre point and hammer in a stake to which a strong line is attached. Use a peg attached to the end of this line to trace out the circumference of your wheel. Then choose a point on this line to mark out a smaller circle to form a centre bed. The line can then be used to plot radii of paths and beds between them. Plan your paths in brick or stone and lay them on a good hardcore/sand base at least 7.5cm (3in) deep. Ensure that the circumference of the wheel is similarly paved.

When planting, consider carefully what the height and spread of the herbs will be at maturity so that you achieve an even balance to prevent lush growth overwhelming the paving and obscuring your design. Trim the plants when necessary to keep your 'wheel' in shape.

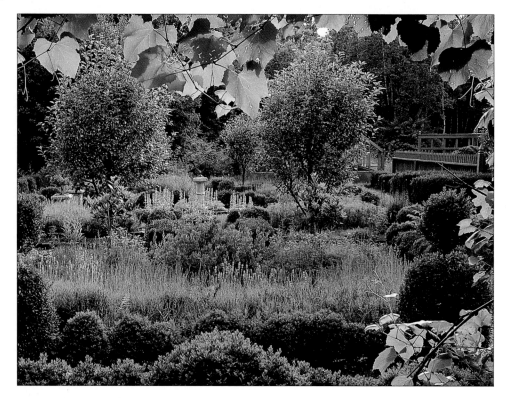

LEFT: *Herb gardens are traditionally centred by some sort of device such as a sundial or armillary sphere, even a piece of sculpture. Since most aromatic herbs need full sunlight, a sundial is an obvious choice.*
RIGHT: *Parterre gardens are part of a formal garden tradition where the variety of herbs is subordinated to their effect as a pattern. This parterre uses* Buxus sempervirens *in diamond shapes filled with Common Germander* Teucrium chamaedrys, *traditionally used in decoction as tonic.*

Herb gardens provide an excellent way of combining traditional design with your own personal ideas. However, perhaps because of the relatively short life of most herbs, few old herb gardens still exist; they are transient phenomena compared to gardens of woody plants. In Britain interesting formal herb gardens can be seen at Knebworth House in Hertfordshire (which has been reconstructed to an original design by Gertrude Jekyll of interlocking circles of brick); at Wisley in Surrey (designed for access by disabled visitors); at Leeds Castle in Kent ('The Culpeper Garden'); at Sissinghurst in Kent (where there is also a beautiful thyme lawn); and at the American Museum, Claverton, Avon (which is delightfully centred by a bee skep). At the Royal Botanic Gardens, Kew, the Queen's Garden has been planted with seventeenth-century plants, many of them labelled with amusing quotations from Gerard's *Herball* as to their uses.

In the USA, herb gardens displaying plants named in the plays and sonnets of Shakespeare are popular. A well-maintained example can be seen at the Brooklyn Botanic Garden and is well worth a visit.

Informal herb gardens are seen less often, though herbs have always been planted informally close to the house in traditional cottage gardens. Indeed, part of the charm of the cottage garden tradition is that of the haphazard associations and arrangements of plants, and there are many people who still prefer to grow their herbs in this delightful way.

Herb gardens are ideal places to site accessories such as bee skeps because of the large number of fragrant herbs which make good nectar and pollen forage. Since herb gardens should be built in full sun, try siting sundials and armillary spheres which now are available as replicas in a range of historic styles. Other ideas for centrepieces include old copper boilers, terracotta or glazed urns, birdbaths, old well-heads, fountains or pieces of sculpture. At Sissinghurst Castle in Kent the herb garden contains a low, shallow stone dish filled with sempervivums which thrive in the heat and good drainage.

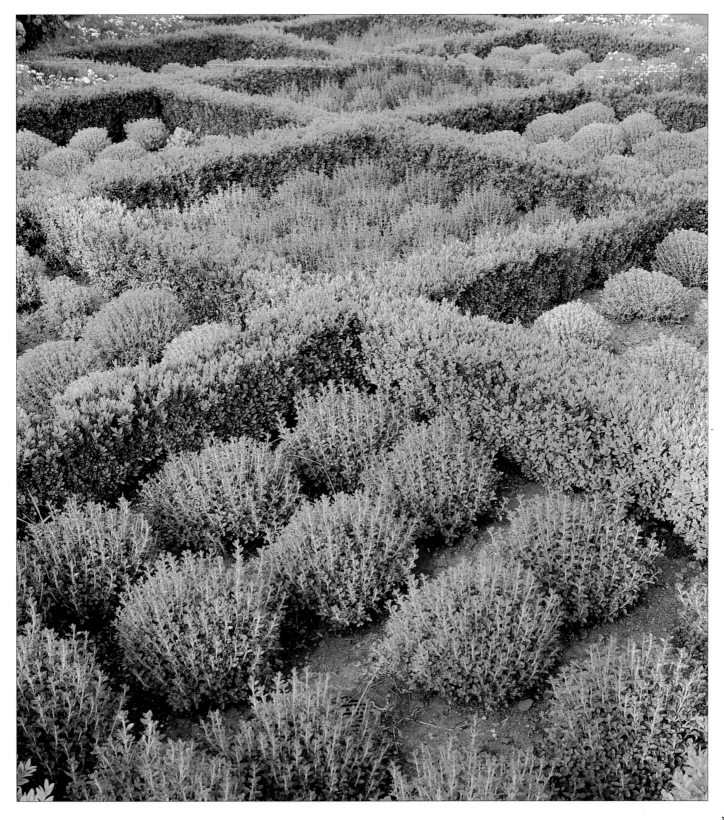

GROWING MEDICINAL PLANTS
FOR ORNAMENT

There is quite a range of plants used either in traditional herbalism or as drug plants in orthodox medicine which are very ornamental in their own right. All of the following species could be used to create an alternative specialist area in your own garden. I would suggest using the woody species such as Hawthorn, Witch Hazel, Elder, *Vitex* and *Rosa* as a structure planting and infill with the perennial species. For extra height you can train the hop onto a tripod of stakes or an ornamental iron column. Leave spaces to sow some of the species which are fast-growing annuals and can be sown outdoors in spring. These include the Opium Poppy, Melilot, the Castor Oil Plant, and the annual *Artemisia*. If you are growing these in a border rather than a central bed, pay attention to the mature height of the plants and grade them down to the shortest in the front.

Achillea millefolium Yarrow
This is a perennial plant native to Britain with feathery foliage and white flattened heads of flowers throughout summer. It grows up to 60cm (2ft) tall and spreads vigorously (some would say it is weedlike). It will grow well at the front of a border. There is also a pink variety called 'Cerise Queen'. Yarrow will seed itself and you will need to be disciplined in confining it. John Parkinson's *Paradisus* of 1629 recommended it for staunching bleeding, and it was used for this purpose in emergency in World War One.

Althaea officinalis Marsh Mallow
This is a perennial plant of moist places that grows rapidly to 90cm–1.2 metres (3–4ft). Its lobed leaves are typical of the mallow family, and the flowers are pink. In herbal medicine the roots and leaves are used in compresses to reduce inflammation. Culpeper also recommended Marsh Mallow for coughs and chest infections. The plant can be grown from spring-sown seed or from cuttings. It will succeed in any soil, but will grow more luxuriantly in rich, moist conditions.

Artemisia annua
This is a plant of the daisy family that you can raise from seed sown direct into the ground in spring. It grows to about 60cm (2ft) and produces attractive feathery leaves and short spikes of insignificant flowers in late summer. It has been used for centuries in China to treat malaria and artemesinin extracted from it is now used to treat cerebral malaria which is resistant to treatment by synthetic drugs.

Centaurium erythraea Centaury
This is really a wild flower of English chalk downlands and needs poor, limy soil to do well. It will grow to 30cm (1ft) in height (often less) and produces panicles of pink flowers on slender stems. This bitter herb has been used in herbal medicine to relieve gout, and to stimulate the liver and digestion.

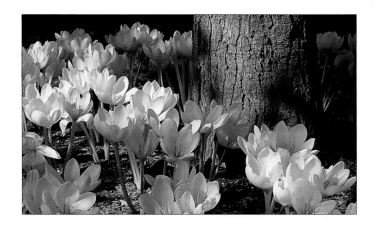

Colchicum autumnale *var.* album, *white Meadow Saffron.*

Colchicum autumnale Meadow Saffron

This is a bulbous plant that flowers in the late summer and early autumn when it produces charming lilac flowers similar to large crocuses on leafless stems. The rather coarse leaves growing up to 30cm (1ft) or more follow in the spring. Plant the large corms in late summer in rich well-drained soil at the front of a border. Meadow Saffron was used in the ancient world for arthritis and it is still used to treat gout. Colchicine extracted from it is one of the chemicals used in genetic and cancer research as it causes chromosomes to double.

Crataegus laevigata Hawthorn

This is a native European deciduous tree species that grows to 7 metres (23ft) high and as much wide. It produces white flowers in late spring and crimson fruits in autumn. It can be grown as a standard tree – or clipped into an excellent hedge if you wish one to enclose or back your medicinal border. In herbal medicine the fruits are used to treat kidney stones (Culpeper recommended it highly) and it has been used in cardiology. Country folk say its smell is a reminder of the Great Plague.

Digitalis lanata Woolly Foxglove

This species is probably less well known than its purple-flowered cousin, but it is the species which is mostly cropped commercially for the digoxin it contains – used in the treatment of weak and irregular heart rhythms. It is a perennial plant, growing to 60–90cm (2–3ft) tall and has downy grey flowers in mid summer. *D. purpurea* is more showy and contains digitoxin. It is not cropped to the same extent by pharmaceutical companies. Both are easily raised from seed sown in the open ground in spring. *D. purpurea* prefers some shade or woodland conditions.

Dryopteris filix-mas Male Fern

This British native fern is useful in providing a soft, green element among flowering plants. Buy it as a plant rather than try the long process of raising the spores. It was once used as a vermifuge; that is, for the eradication of worms.

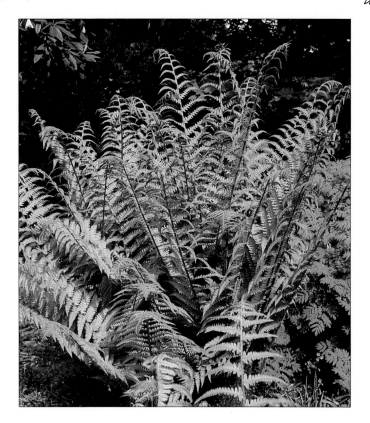

The Male Fern was an effective treatment for tapeworm.

Filipendula ulmaria Meadowsweet

This British native plant really needs a very moist place to do well, but will then charm you with its spikes of creamy flowers with their musky smell of meadowland. If grown well it will reach 45cm (18in). Plant Meadowsweet if you suffer from headaches to remind you that it was in 1835 that salicylic acid was first extracted from this plant. Aspirin (acetyl-salicylic acid) was introduced 64 years later.

Gentiana lutea Yellow Gentian

This European native perennial will shoot up vigorously to 1.2–1.6 metres (4–5ft) producing a spike of yellow star-like flowers. It needs a moist soil and partial shade and is easily raised from seed. The medicinal part of the plant is its thick root, which is used in herbal medicine to stimulate the appetite and tone the digestive system. Culpeper also recommended it for agues and fevers.

THE MYTH OF THE MANDRAKE

This is an extraordinary plant in both its appearance and the myths surrounding its medicinal properties. For this alone it is worth including in any medicinal border.

Mandragora officinarum Mandrake is a plant native to the warmer parts of Europe. It contains the powerful relaxant drug hyoscine in its roots and fruit. In medieval Britain and Europe powerful myths arose about this plant, its wonderful painkilling properties and how it could be collected. It was believed that you would die if you dug it up, because the roots looked like the human body and under the theory of the Doctrine of Signatures (see page 18) this would be akin to doing someone to death. The mandrake would scream in the process. The myth recommended tying a dog to the plant and allowing it to uproot it while the collector would stop his or her ears to drown the sound. It was also believed (erroneously) that mandrake plants were either male or female; illustrations in herbals often show two plants, one appearing like the figure of a man and the other a woman.

Wine of mandrake was used in the sponge given to crucifixion victims to put a merciful end to their agonies.

Although its flowers are nondescript, the fruits of the mandrake (like green tomatoes) provide a wonderful, long-lasting feature at the front of a border, besides giving you the opportunity of telling gripping tales!

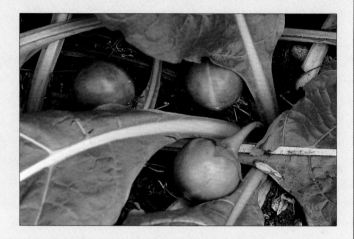

Mandrake fruits last from spring until autumn.

Glycyrrhiza glabra Liquorice
This is a perennial member of the pea family and comes from the Mediterranean where it grows 90cm–1.2 metres (3–4ft) tall. The attractive pale blue flowers are produced in late summer and autumn. Like the Yellow Gentian the medically active part of the plant is the root, which has been traditionally used in herbal medicine for indigestion. The semi-synthetic drug carbenoxalone has been derived from it and is used to treat peptic ulcers.

Hamamelis virginiana Witch Hazel
Witch Hazel is a shrub from eastern North America which produces sweetly scented yellow flowers in autumn as the foliage turns bright yellow. It will grow to 5 metres (16ft) tall and as much wide. Traditionally used by North American Indians to treat skin problems, the astringent bark is recognized in the US *Pharmacopoeia*. It is a charming shrub but needs moist, deep soil.

Humulus lupulus Hop
The climbing hop which forms an essential ingredient in beer has been used for centuries to induce sleep. A vigorous climber (too vigorous for most gardens) it is best grown as its golden-leaved variant *Humulus lupulus* 'Aureus' which is less rampant and highly ornamental, although it rarely produces much flower.

Iris germanica var. *florentina* Orris
The flowering of this pale blue flag iris around Florence is often a sight to behold, and is a remnant of the medieval perfume industry in which the powdered roots were used. Orris was also used to clear bronchial congestion and as snuff. The plants must have full sun. Their rhizomes should be planted just at soil level and firmed in very well. Divide and replant them every three or four years. The flowering spikes reach 90cm (3ft) when they appear in late spring, but are rather short lived.

Inula helenium Elecampane

This is a yellow-flowered daisy that will grow up to 1.5 metres (5ft) in good, moist soil and partial shade. The medicinal part is the root, which is bactericidal and was formerly used in treating tuberculosis. Both Gerard and Culpeper recommended it for all manner of coughs. It can be raised easily from seed.

Melilotus officinalis Melilot

This is an annual member of the pea family with clover-like leaves and profuse yellow flowers. It grows rapidly from seed sown in the open ground in spring, and flowers in early to mid summer. It is best to stake the plant with stout, twiggy branches to stop it flopping over. This is an interesting plant to grow if you are on anticoagulant drugs to combat thrombosis; it was dicoumarol in the hay made from Melilot that was found to cause haemorrhages in cattle and led to the entire idea of anticoagulants such as warfarin.

Oenothera biennis Evening Primrose

This is an American genus and this species is a biennial growing to a good 90cm–1 metre (3–3¹⁄₂ft) in its second year. The pale yellow flowers are very profuse and open (in the evening) successively from early summer to mid autumn, so it is a worthy member of an ornamental medicinal garden. It tolerates any soil but must have full sun. Allow it to seed and you will never be short of seedlings, but you might need to weed out a few that have spread too far. The medicinal part of the plant is the gamma-linolenic acid that is contained in the oil expressed from the seed. This is useful in treating eczema and is used as a dietary supplement to relieve premenstrual tension. Long used by North American Indians it has now been genetically improved as a crop plant.

Papaver somniferum Opium Poppy

This is one of the most beautiful of the annual poppies with silvery-grey leaves and ephemeral flowers in a range of pinks, either single or double-flowered. The flowers are followed by the handsome pods from which the latex is harvested

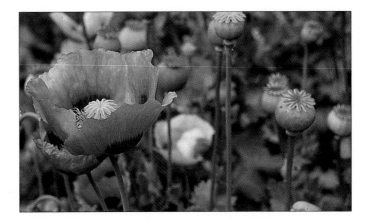

The pods of the opium poppy contain morphine.

to turn into morphine, codeine (or heroin on the black market). There is no restriction on cultivating Opium Poppies in the garden (unlike Cannabis) since they rarely ripen enough to produce the active ingredient. The plant seeds freely and you may need to remove most of the pods before they ripen to restrict self-seeding. Dry them to make excellent indoor decorations.

Podophyllum hexandrum and Podophyllum peltatum
Indian and American Mandrake

These attractive herbaceous perennials need a rich moist soil and some shade. They are useful for providing a display of handsome, brownish leaves and have ephemeral pinkish flowers followed by large scarlet fruits. Use them at the front of a border because neither plant grows to more than 30cm (1ft). Semi-synthetic drugs based on extracts from the roots are used to treat lung, kidney and testicular cancers.

Primula veris Cowslip

This charming spring-flowering British native is a plant for the front of the border. Its leaves expand rapidly in early spring in small rosettes from which the heads of yellow scented flowers emerge. In herbal medicine this plant was used to treat migraine, especially when taken as Cowslip wine, and Culpeper recommended it for acne and other skin eruptions. Modern herbalists still use the flowers to relieve tension headaches.

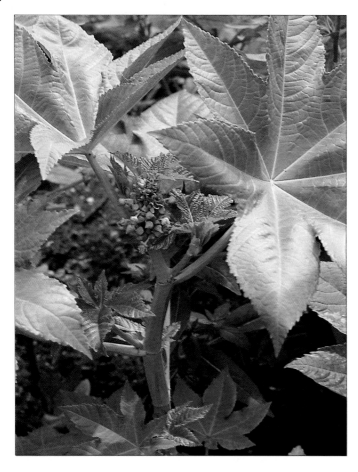

The seed of Ricinus communis *yields Castor Oil.*

Rheum palmatum

This plant is a relative of the common or garden Rhubarb *R. rhaponticum*, and originates from China, where its roots have been used to treat both constipation and dysentery. It is a useful foliage plant to grow for dramatic effect and will easily grow to 1.5 metres (5ft) in good soil, producing handsome panicles of red flowers in mid summer.

Ricinus communis Castor Oil Plant

This is a handsome plant with large, palmate leaves and is often grown as a 'dot' plant; that is, a plant used in bedding schemes as a specimen to give height. It is perennial in areas with a Mediterranean climate, but is best sown from seed each year elsewhere. It will easily grow to 1.2 metres (4ft) in a season. The oil from the seeds is

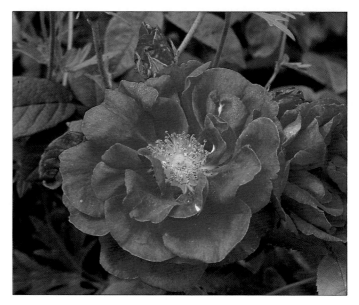

The Apothecaries' Rose was widely used by French druggists.

well known as a drastic remedy for constipation and is very foul tasting. The seedcoat itself (rather than the oil), however, contains the deadly poison ricin. Involved in several murders (including the murder of Bulgarian diplomat Markov by injection from a lethal umbrella point) this plant is sometimes grown for its rather gruesome history! The Victorians loved to grow it in beds of subtropical bedding plants for its exotic effect.

The genus *Rosa*

The main species of rose used medicinally are *R. damascena* Damask Rose and *R. centifolia* Cabbage Rose. Both of these flower once but gloriously, and are used in perfumery and aromatherapy. *R. canina*, the wild English Dog Rose, produces scarlet hips which are used to produce Rose hip syrup, an excellent source of vitamin C. It is rarely planted in gardens (except in wild gardens), however, because of its brief flowering period. *R. gallica* was used to produce astringent rose water, while *R. gallica* 'Officinalis' became known as the Apothecaries' Rose because it was used widely in French folk medicine to treat sore throats and diarrhoea. *R. gallica* 'Officinalis' has a rather harsh red and white flower said to symbolize the settlement of

THE PLANT ORIGINS OF SOME MAJOR MODERN DRUGS

There are a number of important drugs that owe their origin directly to a plant. In some cases the active ingredient from the plant is used directly (artemisinin, digoxin, vincristine, atropine and morphine). In others, the plant ingredient provides the basis upon which a part-synthetic drug is developed (etoposide). In a few cases discovery of the active ingredient has led to the development of a synthetic drug (contraceptive steroids are now synthesized rather than extracted from yams). Chemists have also copied how a plant's secondary compounds work and have developed a more reliable synthetic drug (dicoumarol). Biochemists are now much more successful at isolating compounds from plants.

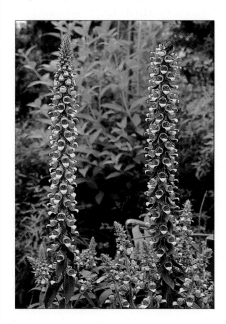

Digitalis lanata is cropped for the digoxin it contains.

Drug	Medical use	Plant source
Amiodarone	For heartbeat irregularity.	*Ammi visnaga*
Artemisinin	For malaria.	*Artemisia annua*
Aspirin	As a painkiller.	*Filipendula ulmaria* Meadowsweet
Atropine	To stimulate the heart during heart attack.	*Atropa belladonna* Deadly Nightshade
Carbenoxalone	For peptic ulcer.	*Glycyrrhiza glabra* Liquorice
Cocaine	As a painkiller.	*Erythroxylum coca* Coca
Codeine	As a painkiller.	*Papaver somniferum* Opium Poppy
Colchicine	For gout.	*Colchicum autumnale* Meadow Saffron
Dicoumarol	As an anticoagulant to prevent thrombosis.	*Melilotus officinalis* Melilot
Digoxin	To strengthen and normalize heartbeat.	*Digitalis lanata* Woolly Foxglove
Epogam	For eczema.	*Oenothera biennis* Evening Primrose
Etoposide	For various cancers.	*Podophyllum hexandrum* Indian Mandrake
Hyoscine and Hyoscyamine	As a relaxant before major anaesthesia; for motion sickness.	*Mandragora officinarum* Mandrake, but commercially from *Duboisia myoporoides*
Lignocaine	As a local anaesthesic.	*Hordeum vulgare* Barley
Methoxsalen	For skin cancer, psoriasis and vitiligo.	*Ammi majus*
Morphine	As an excellent painkiller.	*Papaver somniferum* Opium Poppy
Nifedipine	For angina and hypertension.	*Ammi visnaga*
Physostigmine	For paralysis in myasthenia gravis; glaucoma.	*Physostigma venenosum* Ordeal Bean
Pilocarpine	For glaucoma.	*Pilocarpus microphyllus* Jaborandi
Quinidine	For irregular heartbeat.	*Cinchona* sp. Quinine
Quinine	For malaria and muscle cramps.	*Cinchona* sp. Quinine
Salicin	As a painkiller and anti-rheumatic.	*Salix* sp. Willow
Steroids (including contraceptives)	To reduce inflammation and to prevent conception.	*Agave sisalana* Sisal and *Dioscorea* sp. Yam
Theophylline	To reduce excess blood formation after kidney transplantation; as a diuretic.	*Camellia sinensis* Tea
Tubocurarine	As a muscle relaxant.	*Chondrodendron tomentosum* Curare
Vincristine and Vinblastine	For leukaemia and Hodgkin's disease.	*Catharanthus roseus* Rosy Periwinkle

the medieval Wars of the Roses and is therefore a symbol of peace. All these roses need full sun.

Sambucus nigra Elder

Elder is a European shrub that may grow to 8 metres (27ft) but is more often seen in hedgerows at about 4 or 5 metres (13–16ft). It is well known for its flat heads of creamy white heavily scented flowers in early summer that can be made into syrup, wine or 'Elderflower champagne'. Elder-flower water was once listed in the British *Pharma-copoeia* as a base for skin and eye lotions and was recommended by Culpeper, who also promoted Elderflower root as a purgative. The flowers are used in modern herbal medicine for fevers. Elder needs a moist soil and is a good plant for the wild garden where its habit of seeding profusely and providing fruits for birds is welcome. Do not plant it in a border unless you are prepared to hoe out its seedlings.

Scutellaria lateriflora Skullcap

This (and other species of skullcap) were long thought to help 'head' diseases through the Doc-trine of Signatures (see page 18), but are nowa-days used in herbal medicine for nervous exhaustion. This species grows to 60–90cm (2–3ft) and needs moist soil. The flowers are blue and helmet shaped like medieval skullcaps.

Symphytum officinale Comfrey

Keep this plant for the wild garden where it can spread without becoming an invasive weed. It grows to 60–90cm (2–3ft) with hairy leaves and arching sprays of flowers of cream and purplish-pink. Long known as 'knitbone', Comfrey was pre-scribed by Culpeper for bruises, ruptures and fractures when the roots were applied as a poultice. The allantoin it contains is still used nowadays in salves. In Australia, the cultivation and medicinal use of Comfrey is subject to strict legislation.

Tanacetum parthenium Feverfew

This member of the daisy family grows to about 90cm (3ft) and produces great masses of small white flowers from early summer onwards. The golden-leaved variety is useful to add foliage colour to a border and there is also a very orna-mental double-flowered form. Feverfew was used to quell fevers and both Culpeper and Gerard rec-ommended it as an anti-depressant. Today it is used to dilate the blood vessels in migraine attacks and various forms of it have been used in trials at the Chelsea Physic Garden under funding by the Migraine Trust. It is best not taken fresh (to avoid mouth ulcers) and should always be avoid-ed in pregnancy. Feverfew is easily raised from seed and will spread itself if excess seedlings are not weeded out.

Valeriana officinalis Valerian

The medicinal Valerian is a perennial plant found throughout temperate Europe and North America where it will grow to 1.2 metres (4ft). The flowers are white, tinged pink – as opposed to the Red Valerian *Centranthus ruber* which has no medicinal value at all – but it is in the roots where the value of the plant as a sedative is found. Obtain a plant as it is slow from seed, and do not plant it if you have cats, unless you want them to be transported into paroxysms of delight (as with Catmint) and have enough plants to withstand their rolling in it.

Veratrum viride Green Hellebore

Not a true hellebore at all, this plant is a stately member of the lily family with elegant pleated leaves. The flowering spike of yellowish flowers will rise to 2 metres (6½ft) by mid summer if it is planted in rich soil the previous autumn. Plant young plants in partial shade or the heat of the midday sun will disfigure the leaves by scorching them. The medicinal part of the plant is the black root which contains alkaloids once used to treat high blood pressure.

Verbena officinalis Vervain

Vervain is an annual found throughout Europe where it grows to 1 metre (3ft) and produces small purplish flowers. Like most species named 'officinale' it was a herb sold in shops for medici-nal purposes, and had a long connection with sorcery. Gerard dismissed these uses and Culpeper recommended it for stomach and digestive problems. Nowadays it is used in herbalism as a tonic. Vervain is easy to grow from seed in any soil, but prefers sun.

Viola odorata Sweet Violet

This is a small perennial well suited to the front of a shady border in a humus-rich soil where it will spread by runners. It produces sweetly scented flowers in early spring, purple in the type and white in the variety 'Alba'. In modern herbal medicine it is used to treat inflammation, as it was in the days of Gerard and Culpeper. It contains methyl salicylate, similar to aspirin.

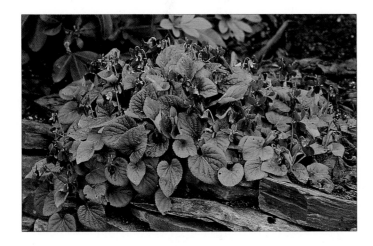

Viola odorata is used in modern and ancient herbalism.

Viola tricolor Heartsease

This is a pretty and very free-flowering annual for a sunny place at the front of a border. The flowers are purple, white and yellow and, though small, are produced continuously through the summer. Traditionally the flowers have been used in cordials for heart complaints, the top two lobes of the flowers being reminiscent of the upper lobes of the heart under the theory of the Doctrine of Signatures (see page 18).

Vitex agnus-castus Chaste Berry

This is a deciduous shrub from Mediterranean areas and can only be cultivated in very warm gardens, preferably trained against a wall for extra protection. It comes into leaf very late, often not until early summer, and produces its spikes of pale violet flowers in late summer or early autumn. The berries are only produced in very warm areas and ripen late in mid autumn. *Vitex* is used in modern herbalism to affect the pituitary gland and assist with premenstrual tension, menopausal problems and hormonal imbalances.

Medicinal plants to grow indoors or in the conservatory

Camellia sinensis Tea

Tea plants are sometimes available to grow as conservatory plants. Like most of the tender camellias they need minimal heat. Just keep them frost free, in a moisture-retentive compost and provide light shade and they will reward you with small white flowers with golden stamens. The theophylline in tea is used in treating kidney transplant patients.

Capsicum frutescens Cayenne or Chilli Pepper

These make good plants to grow on a sunny windowsill and can be raised from seed sown in mid spring. The plant forms a small bush (especially if the stems are pinched back as they grow), and produce white flowers followed by large fruits that ripen to a bright red. These can be diced and used in Mexican dishes. Cayenne is used in modern herbalism to improve blood circulation.

Carica papaya Pawpaw or Papaya

This is fun to grow as a pot plant from its knobbly little seeds and produces attractive palmate leaves. However, it is unlikely to fruit unless you have a large conservatory. The fruit contains the digestive enzyme papain, which is excellent for sensitive, upset stomachs. Papaya is a wonderful fruit to eat in the morning after a rich meal the night before.

Catharanthus roseus Rosy Periwinkle

This is often sold as a pot plant, either in its pink form or in the varieties 'Alba' (a large-flowered pure white) or 'Ocellata' (a white flower with a central pink eye). You can also grow the plant from seed and it will flower all the year round, although the flowers have the curious habit of being smaller in the winter. It is wise to renew your stock by taking cuttings in spring as the plants can become lanky and do not respond well to being pruned back. The alkaloids this pretty plant contains have probably helped tens of thousands of children suffering from leukaemia.

Gelsemium sempervirens Carolina Jasmine
This evergreen climber from the southern USA needs to be grown in a warm conservatory, preferably planted in a bed of rich soil. It produces its showy yellow flowers in spring. The root is used medicinally in homoeopathy, and has also been used to treat migraine and neuralgia.

Quassia amara
This is a tropical American tree which is occasionally available as a conservatory plant, as it will flower even as a young cutting. The leaves are unusual in having winged stalks with red midribs and the flowers are scarlet. This plant needs to be grown in a warm conservatory and is best in a bed of rich soil. Its bitter bark is used as a tonic and is used, along with the root, against dysentery.

Senna alexandrina Senna
Senna is a shrubby tree that can be grown from seed, providing you soak it in hot water for twenty-four hours before sowing. A member of the pea family, it will produce its yellow flowers even as a small plant and may even set the pods favoured in purgative medicine.

Zingiber officinale Ginger
Ginger can be grown as a foliage pot plant from rhizomes, providing you plant them when they are plump and fresh. They need a rich soil and a warm windowsill where they will produce thin leafy shoots that give a fragrance when bruised. Do not hope for flowers as long cycles of vegetative propagation seem to have reduced this plant's ability to produce them. Ginger has been shown to be very effective against travel sickness and morning sickness in pregnancy.

THE BACH FLOWER REMEDIES

○

Edward Bach was an English physician who practised as a homoeopath in London during the 1920s. He developed a system of remedies based on thirty-seven *wild* plants, using tinctures prepared from them by infusion or by boiling. His concern was to identify cures for the psychological states of individuals that depleted the immune system.

In some ways his emphasis looked forward to the contemporary concern with the effect of the mind on the body. In others it looked back at the medieval Doctrine of Signatures where the appearance or habit of the plant was thought to indicate what it would cure.

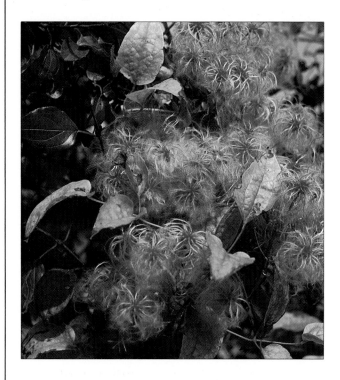

Clematis vitalba is the Bach remedy used for dreamers.

Botanical name	Common name	Used to treat
Aesculus × carnea	Red Chestnut	Fear for others.
Aesculus hippocastanum	White Chestnut	Worry, with an over-active mind.
Aesculus hippocastanum (bud)	White Chestnut	Slowness in learning.
Agrimonia eupatoria	Agrimony	Worry, when hidden by a cheerful façade.
Bromus ramosus	Wild Oat	Lack of direction.
Calluna vulgaris	Ling	Fear of loneliness in those self-absorbed.
Carpinus betulus	Hornbeam	Fear of lack of strength in daily duties.
Castanea sativa	Sweet Chestnut	Anguish in those exhausted.
Centaurium umbellatum	Centaury	For those who give in too much to the demands of others.
Ceratostigma willmottianum	Plumbago	Indecision.
Cichorium intybus	Chicory	Possessiveness, in those critical of others.
Clematis vitalba	Old Man's Beard	For those who are not rooted in the present and tend to dream.
Fagus sylvatica	Beech	Intolerance.
*Gentiana amarella**	Felwort	Self-doubt.
Helianthemum nummularium	Rock Rose	Terror.
Hottonia palustris	Water Violet	Reticence, over self-reliance.
Ilex aquifolium	Holly	For jealousy, envy, desire for revenge.
Impatiens glandulifera	Impatiens	Irritability, impatience.
Juglans regia	Walnut	For those distracted by others from their own life aims.
Larix decidua	Larch	Lack of self-confidence and fear of failure.
Lonicera caprifolium	Honeysuckle	For those who look back too much to happier days.
Malus pumila	Crab Apple	For those who feel unclean.
Mimulus guttatus	Monkey Flower	Phobias.
Olea europaea	Olive	Mental prostration.
Ornithogalum umbellatum	Star of Bethlehem	Shock.
Pinus sylvestris	Scots Pine	Self-reproach.
Populus tremula	Aspen	Fears: source unknown.
Prunus cerasifera	Cherry Plum	Fears of insanity or senility.
Quercus robur	English Oak	Depression, in those who battle courageously.
Rosa canina	Wild Rose	Apathy.
Salix alba var. *vitellina*	Yellow Willow	For bitterness and resentment.
Scleranthus annuus	Scleranthus	Indecision, without resort to advice.
Sinapsis arvensis	Mustard	Severe, unexplainable depression.
Ulex europaeus	Gorse	Despair.
Ulmus procera	English Elm	For those who feel overburdened by responsibility.
Verbena officinalis	Vervain	Strain in those who are energetic but have fixed ideas.
Vitis vinifera	Grape Vine	Dominance, over-forcefulness.

*There is doubt over which species Bach identified.
For more information contact The Dr Edward Bach Centre, Mount Vernon, Sotwell, Wallingford, Oxon OX10 0PZ, England.

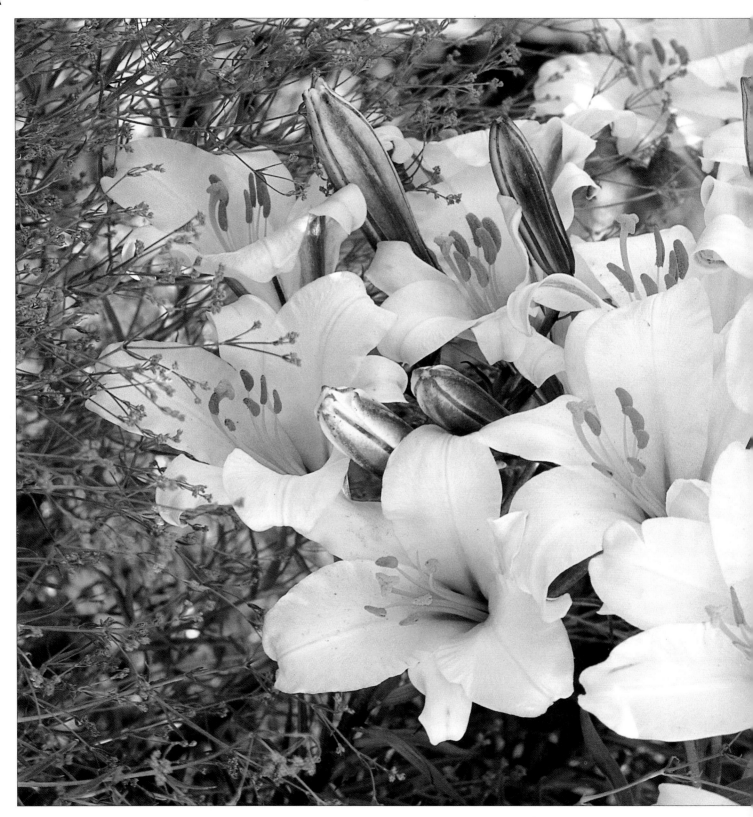

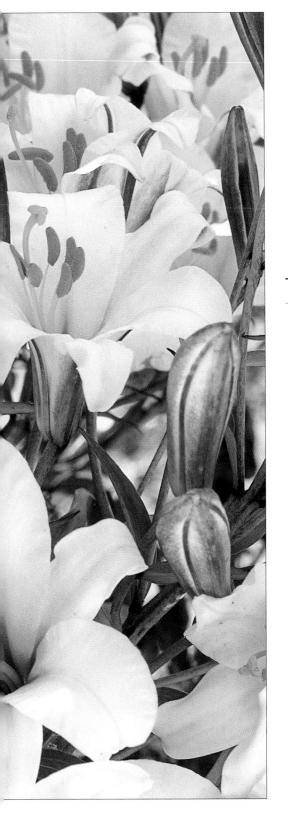

CHAPTER THREE

THE SENSES AWAKENED

○

Experience enhanced

Plants give us pleasure and can bring healing through our five senses, either physically or more indirectly via memories and moods. Herbs can enhance your enjoyment and delight in the taste of good food, with added pleasure if you have grown them yourself. The joy of colour in a garden needs skill to contrive successfully, especially as it involves designing with the fourth dimension, time. Done well, it can affect mood beneficially and therapeutically. Equally soothing are the sounds that surround you in the garden. Perfume, on the other hand, stimulates memory and can be used to evoke happy times to heal us psychologically. There can also be great pleasure in a well-designed scented garden, while aromatherapists contend that the oils of certain plants heal us directly. Then there are plants which are a joy to touch, plants whose texture itself is a pleasure which can surprise and delight us. All we need is to be prepared to have our senses awakened. Some key species that appeal to the senses are illustrated on pages 70–71.

Lilium regale is a Chinese species which produces an overpowering scent, especially strong at night.

PLANTS TO DELIGHT OUR SENSES

○

Here are plants to perfume our rooms and gardens, enrich our palates, soothe us with the sounds of the wind through their leaves and delight us by their textures or by the joy of their colour.

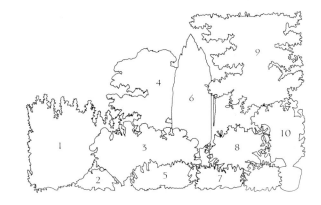

1. Rosemary *Rosmarinus officinalis* produces an invigorating oil much used in aromatherapy as well as in cookery. The shrub is rather tender and needs a warm, protected spot.

2. The Peppermint Geranium *Pelargonium tomentosum* delights the nose by the scent released when the soft leaves are touched. This plant needs full protection from frost.

3. *Rosa centifolia* is one of the species from which rose oil is distilled and used in rose water and in aromatherapy. Plant in the winter in fertile soil.

4. The gum *Eucalyptus globosus* is the main species used for the production of the expectorant eucalyptus oil. This species needs shelter. It can be cut hard back in spring to keep it as a bushy shrub.

5. Lavender is cropped from *Lavandula angustifolia*, the species with no tinge of camphor. Lavender oil is relaxing and relieves headaches. Plant in spring in fairly infertile soil in full sun.

6. Juniper *Juniperus communis* produces an oil used in aromatherapy as well as the berries used to flavour gin. A tough conifer, it needs full sun and is best planted in early autumn.

7. Basil *Ocimum basilicum* is the finest herb for use with tomatoes and Provençal dishes and is the essential ingredient of pesto (see page 76). It must be raised annually from seed and is very frost-tender.

8. The Tobacco Plant *Nicotiana alata* releases its scent only in the evening. Raise it from seed sown in the spring.

9. The Honeysuckle *Lonicera japonica* 'Halliana' is one of the most sweetly fragrant of the genus. Plant it where you can enjoy the wafts of scent.

10. The Arabian Jasmine *Jasminum sambac* is used to flavour jasmine tea and is a highly ornamental pot plant, especially as the double-flowered form 'Duke of Tuscany'.

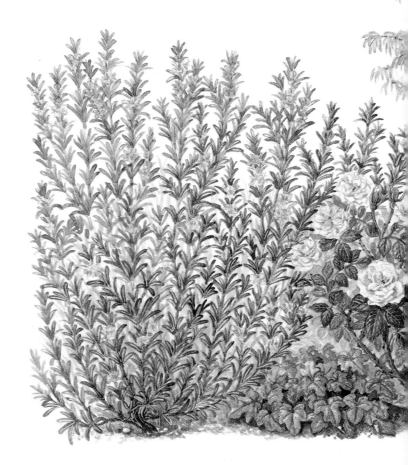

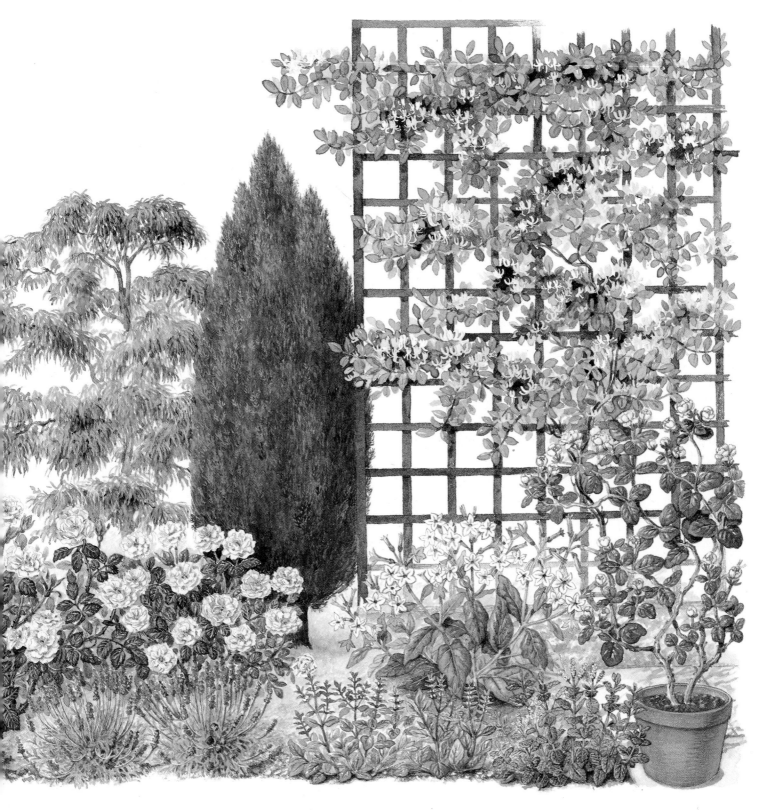

THE MAINSTAY CULINARY HERBS

○

In cookery, herbs are used to bring out and emphasize the natural flavours of foods or to complement them. By tradition, certain herbs are used with certain dishes, sometimes to aid digestion, and are sometimes strongly linked with national or regional cuisines. Try using them in unconventional ways, however, and you may reawaken your taste buds!

Herbs also make attractive garnishes, adding visual enjoyment to the dish.

Angelica *Angelica archangelica*

Candy young stems to decorate cakes. Cook roots and stems.

This biennial herb needs to be grown in slight shade. Sow seed in late summer, and thin seedlings to 15cm (6in) apart.

Anise *Pimpinella anisum*

Use anise leaves in salads and fruit salads and with shellfish dishes for a mild aniseed taste. Anise seeds are useful in biscuits and cakes.

Sow seed in open ground after the risk of frost is past. Thin to 15cm (6in) apart. Gather in autumn and dry the seedheads.

Basil

SWEET BASIL *Ocimum basilicum*
Basil is the finest herb for use in Mediterranean dishes, especially with tomatoes.

Sow the seeds under glass in mid spring and do not plant out until all risk of frost is past. Ensure the compost is well drained.

'MINIMUM' BUSH BASIL
Ocimum basilicum
Grow and use as sweet basil. This variety is excellent for pot culture due to its bushy habit.

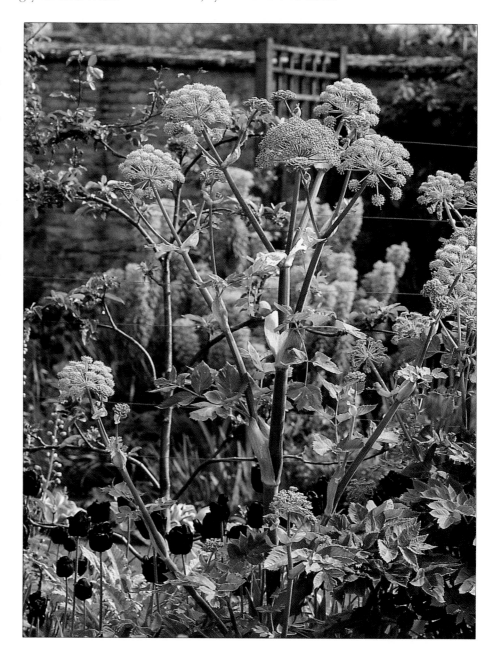

RIGHT: Angelica produces succulent stems, attractive in cake decoration.

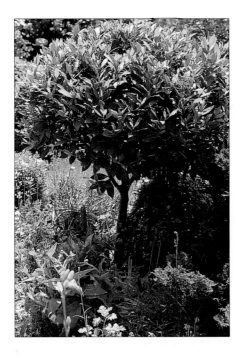

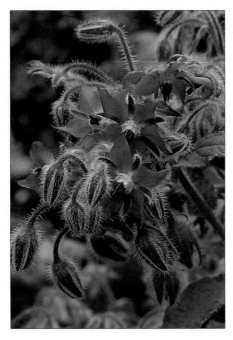

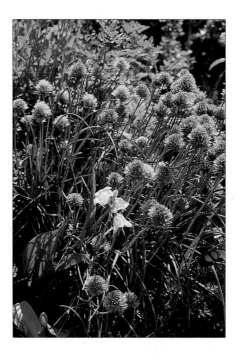

Bay produces leaves abundantly.

Borage flowers can change to pink.

Clumps of chives can increase rapidly.

Bay *Laurus nobilis*

Add bay leaves to soups, stews and to the water in which fish is poached or lightly boiled.

Plant a young plant in full sun and increase by cuttings.

Bergamot *Monarda didyma*

Add bergamot leaves and flowers to green salads, fruit salads, fruit cups and jellies.

Plant as a young plant in rich soil in light shade. Increase by division in spring or autumn.

Borage *Borago officinalis*

Young borage leaves can be chopped into salads. Use the flowers to decorate fruit punches, where they will change colour from blue to pink.

Sow seed in poorish soil in spring and in full sun.

Caraway *Carum carvi*

Use caraway seed to flavour pork dishes or in cooked cabbage. It is also traditionally used on biscuits and breads.

Sow seed in the open ground in early summer in light soil in full sun. Harvest the seedheads in the autumn and dry them indoors. They are best in the second year.

Chervil *Anthriscus cereifolium*

Use chopped chervil leaves in salads, soups and sauces. Chervil is traditionally used in egg dishes and as a vegetable garnish.

Sow successively throughout the spring and early summer in well-drained soil in partial shade.

Chives *Allium schoenoprasum*

Chop chives into salads, omelettes and soups. Blend them with sour cream as a topping.

Sow seed in spring. Thereafter propagate by division in spring every few years.

Coriander *Coriandrum sativum*

Use coriander leaves in curries and in green salads. The seed is also used in curries and to spice bland vegetables such as cauliflower. When ground it is good in cakes and biscuits.

Sow successively in light ground from spring until early summer if grown for its leaves. Leave the first sowings to mature for their seed.

Cumin *Cuminum cyminum*

Use cumin in stews, soups and curries and for flavouring cakes and biscuits. Cumin is used extensively in Indian, Mexican and Lebanese cooking, and in confectionary.

Sow in rich soil in early summer

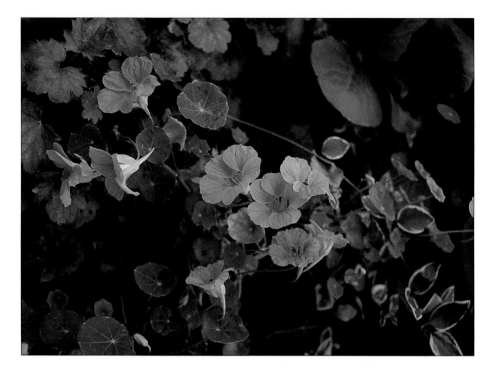

Nasturtium flowers are edible and peppery.

in full sun. Harvest when the plant has died back and dry the seed indoors. Bottle and store to use in cooking as required.

Dill *Anethum graveolens*

Dill is very useful chopped into fish sauces and into salads. The seed is commonly used in the pickling of cucumber and gherkins.

Sow seed in spring and successionally into summer. Dill needs to grow in a rich, moist soil in sun to reach its full potential.

Fennel *Foeniculum vulgare*

Add fennel to fish sauces or as a garnish. The seeds can be used in dough mixes, and they can be chewed as a digestive.

Sow seed in moist, rich soil in spring in sun.

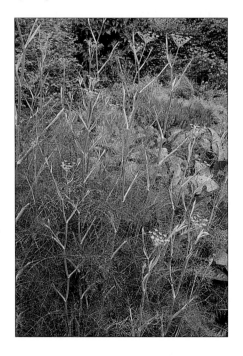

Fennel is a fine-foliaged herb.

FLORENCE FENNEL (*F.v.* var. *dulce*)

The swollen stem bases of Florence fennel can be cooked as a vegetable or chopped into salads.

This plant only matures in very warm gardens.

Lemon Verbena *Aloysia triphylla*

Use lemon verbena leaves in fruit salads, fruit drinks or punch for a strong lemon flavour. They can also be used to flavour custards, ice cream and sorbets.

Plant out after all frost is past if you wish to buy in a plant. Take cuttings in early summer for further stock. Plant in full sun at the foot of a protected wall and protect from frost in winter.

Lovage *Levisticum officinale*

Use lovage leaves in soups and stews, or use young stems as a cooked vegetable. Add leaves to salads and omelettes for a really novel flavour.

Sow seed in late summer. Thereafter propagate by division. This herb requires a lot of space.

Marjoram *Origanum onites*

Add marjoram to meat dishes, and liberally to potatoes when frying.

Sow seed in spring in a well-drained, rich soil.

SWEET MARJORAM *O. marjorana*

Add this variety of pot marjoram to meat dishes.

Sow seed under glass in early spring and plant out in late spring.

WILD MARJORAM OR OREGANO
O. vulgare

This herb has a stronger flavour than the other varieties of pot marjoram. It is good for drying and using in all Mediterranean dishes.

Sow seed in spring.

Mint

APPLE MINT *Mentha suaveolens rotundifolia*
PEPPERMINT *Mentha piperita*
SPEARMINT *Mentha spicata*

Mint is traditionally used as a sauce with lamb dishes, peas and potatoes. It can also be used with all other vegetables.

Plant all varieties of mint in moist soil in partial shade on its own or in a part-sunken bottomless container (all mints are invasive and need to be contained).

Nasturtium *Tropaeolum majus*

Use nasturtium leaves in green salads for their peppery flavour. The flowers add colour to a salad and they can be eaten as well.

Sow seed in poor soil in full sun in early summer.

Parsley *Petroselinum crispum*

Use parsley in green salads, sauces and especially in fish dishes.

Sow in the open ground in spring. Thin and do not try to transplant. Keep well watered.

FRENCH PARSLEY
Use French parsley where strong parsley flavour is required.

Purslane *Portulaca oleracea*

Use young purslane leaves in green salads or cook the young growth and eat with butter like asparagus.

Sow seed in poor soil in full sun in early summer.

Rosemary *Rosmarinus officinalis*

Rosemary is traditionally used in lamb dishes but is also good with pork and fish. Use it to flavour fruit cups and also in mulled wine.

Plant a young plant in poor soil and full sun in early summer. Propagate from cuttings in late summer to increase stock. Protect the plant from frost and particularly from cold, drying winds. Obtain dwarf varieties for pot culture.

Sage *Salvia officinalis*

Use sage in onion stuffing, with roast or stewed meats, in pea soups and in fruit drinks.

Sow seed under glass in spring. Plant out in a sunny place with well-drained soil.

S. OFFICINALIS *'Purpurascens'* AND
S. OFFICINALIS *'Tricolor'*
These varieties may be used in the same dishes as *S. officinalis* but they have less flavour.

Propagate from cuttings in late spring or early summer.

Savory *Satureja hortensis*

Use savory with meat, egg or fish dishes and in soups, bean dishes, stews and casseroles.

Sow seed in open ground in late spring or early summer.

WINTER SAVORY *S. montana*
Use when Summer savory is not available for a milder taste.

Grow as for Summer savory. Will overwinter unlike Summer savory.

Sweet Cicely *Myrrhis odorata*

Sow in the open ground in spring, in moist soil and partial shade.

Use Sweet Cicely to sweeten tart fruit during cooking, or in omelettes, salads and fruit salads as an alternative to cane or beet sugar.

Tarragon

FRENCH TARRAGON
Artemisia dracunculus

Tarragon is good in fish dishes and with chicken. Use it to flavour white sauces and vinegar.

Sow seed under glass in early spring. Plant out when frost is past, then propagate by cuttings. Cut down and mulch in winter.

RUSSIAN TARRAGON
Artemisia dracunculoides
This variety has a very inferior flavour but is much hardier.

It requires no winter protection.

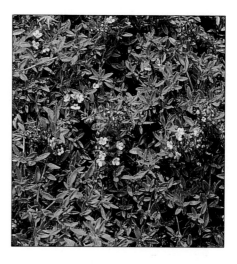

Thymus herba-borona, caraway thyme.

Thyme *Thymus vulgaris*

Use thyme sparingly with meat or fish dishes, soups and casseroles and in stuffings.

Sow in open ground in spring.

LEMON THYME *T. citriodorus*
Use where a milder thyme flavour is required and in stuffings. Also useful to give a lemon flavour in fruit salads and sweets.

Propagate by cuttings in spring.

SOME DELICIOUS RECIPES WITH HERBS

I n the Middle Ages many herbs and spices were used to disguise the flavour of tainted meat, just as strewing herbs were used to cover offensive smells. Today herbs are used to enhance natural flavours, and the following recipes suggest some unusual combinations.

PESTO BASIL SAUCE

1 large bunch basil (or in winter 1 large bunch of parsley and 2 to 3 teaspoons dried basil)
8 tablespoons olive oil
40g (1½oz) grated Parmesan cheese
40g (1½oz) pine kernels
2 cloves crushed garlic

Liquidize the herbs with the garlic, pine kernels, Parmesan and olive oil. Blend at medium speed to produce a soft purée. Add salt to taste.

This serves four when mixed with spaghetti (or other pasta). You can increase the quantities to produce a sauce that can be kept in a jar for several weeks (providing it is refrigerated) and used as required on pasta or to mix into vinaigrette dressing.

RAVIGOTE BUTTER

Butter flavoured with herbs makes a tasty addition to baked potatoes or hot vegetables or as a garnish for cold savoury dishes. Use about 200g (½lb) butter.

1 teaspoon chervil
1 teaspoon chives
1 teaspoon parsley
1 teaspoon tarragon
1 tablespoon chopped shallot

Use fresh herbs if available. Wrap the herbs in muslin. Blanch for three minutes in boiling water. Drain the bag and cool in cold water before wringing out. Blanch the shallots, then blend them together with the herbs. Mix the paste with the butter.

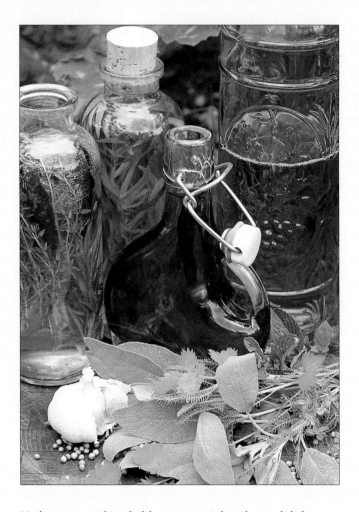

Herb vinegars identified by a sprig rather than a label.

HERB VINEGARS

Herb vinegars are made simply by infusing the herb's aroma into hot vinegar. Chop about ten tablespoons of the herb (basil, salad burnet, dill and tarragon are the usual herb vinegars made) and pour over 150ml (¼ pint) of boiling vinegar. Crush the herb into the vinegar and then add a further 300ml (½ pint) of cold vinegar. Seal into a bottle and shake it every few days for two weeks. Then strain and rebottle.

TOMATO WITH MOZZARELLA VINAIGRETTE

5 large beefsteak-type tomatoes, well ripe
100g (4oz) of sheep or buffalo mozzarella in water
5 or 6 large sprigs of fresh chopped basil
1 mild, thinly sliced onion
3 tablespoons wine vinegar
A little sugar
Salt and pepper
1 teaspoon Dijon mustard
2 cloves garlic, crushed
3 tablespoons olive oil

Mix the sugar, salt and pepper, mustard and crushed garlic into the wine vinegar. Add the oil and mix well. Leave to stand for an hour. Slice the tomatoes onto a plate, then add the sliced onion. Slice the mozzarella over them and cover with the basil. Stir the vinaigrette dressing and pour over the salad.

HERB PUDDING

This is a classic English dish seldom seen.

50g (2oz) pearl barley
100g (4oz) young nettle shoots
100g (4oz) sorrel or young spinach
One bunch spring onions
25g (1oz) parsley
20g (³⁄₄oz) chopped herbs – use a mixture of
marjoram, summer savory, tarragon, dill,
chervil and salad burnet
Salt and black pepper
1 egg

Soak the barley in cold water for four hours, then drain it. Wash the other vegetable ingredients and mix them into the barley along with the chopped herbs. Add salt and pepper. Turn the mixture into a strainer lined with muslin and tie it securely. Simmer the pudding for an hour in water. Drain the pudding and open out into a basin or dish. Beat in the egg and add further salt and pepper to taste. Bake for fifteen minutes in a preheated oven at 180°C (350°F) (Gas Mark 4). The pudding can be eaten on its own or with a meat accompaniment.

LEEKS VINAIGRETTE

Use the vinaigrette recipe (left) and pour it over drained cooked leeks while still hot. Allow the dish to cool and serve lightly chilled.

FENNEL AND LOVAGE SOUP

1 head of Florence fennel
900 ml (1¹⁄₂ pint) chicken stock
1 tablespoon lemon juice
Salt and black pepper
2 tablespoons chopped lovage

Wash the fennel well and slice thinly into a saucepan. Add the stock, bring to the boil, and simmer for about thirty minutes. Strain the soup. Reheat, adding salt, pepper and lemon juice to taste. Stir in the lovage a few minutes before serving.

PEA SOUP WITH SAGE

200g (¹⁄₂ lb) dried green peas
300ml (¹⁄₂ pint) chicken stock
300ml (¹⁄₂ pint) single cream
Salt and black pepper
2 tablespoons finely chopped sage

Cover the peas with boiling water and leave to soak overnight. Cook the peas in water until soft and then purée them in a blender. Add the stock and most of the cream and blend. Add salt and pepper to taste and then the sage. Reheat (do not boil) and serve topped with a swirl of cream.

SOLE WITH CORIANDER

4 pieces of filleted sole (plaice can also be used)
4 tablespoons milk
Salt and black pepper
1 knob of butter
7 or 8 sprigs coriander leaves

Place the fish in a shallow baking dish and cover with milk. Add the knob of butter, add salt and black pepper, then cover the fish with the coriander leaves. Cover the dish and bake in a preheated oven at 200°C (400°F) (Gas Mark 6) for twenty minutes.

DRYING AND STORING HERBS

A good crop of herbs can be preserved for use during the winter by drying, freezing or salting down. It is certainly worth doing this for any of the Mediterranean herbs which really need the summer's heat to produce their full flavour and languish if grown in pots on the windowsill in winter in a misguided attempt to prolong summer's yield.

Drying

The herbs that dry best are thyme, rosemary, bay, marjoram and sage. Pick herbs on a dry morning when the dew has evaporated, and choose growth that is in bud but has not yet produced flowers. You can dry the sprigs in several ways. Either hang them up to dry in a warm, airy place out of direct sunlight, or lay them on a tray covered with muslin for a few days until they are dry but retain their greenness. You can use the warming drawer of an oven, or an airing cupboard.

When the herbs are dry, wrap them whole in paper and store in a drawer or a dry (but dark) larder. You can also crumble them up to save space, discard the woodier stems and then bottle them. Keep the bottles in a dark place or use bottles with darkened glass as light will destroy the flavour of the herbs. Do not leave sprigs of herbs hanging up for any length of time; they may look decorative but the herbs will dry to a dusty, tasteless condition if their flavour is not sealed.

Freezing

Another way of preserving herbs is to freeze them. This is a particularly good method for parsley, fennel and dill which do not dry well. Tarragon sprigs also freeze well. When freezing large-leaved basil, pick individual leaves and freeze them in small freezer bags.

If you have a large ice-making compartment you can produce a ready supply of herb ice cubes by chopping the herbs, adding a little water and freezing the mixtures. Remember to label the ice cube trays. If you eat a lot of grilled meat rather than soups, sauces or stews you can mix the herbs in butter and then freeze the mixture to add to a grill when needed (see page 76).

Salting

Basil leaves are rather fleshy and do not dry well, so the best way of preserving them (apart from freezing) is to salt them. Add salt in layers and then cover the leaves with olive or grapeseed oil. This will preserve basil for up to four weeks and when mixed with vinegar, garlic and black pepper makes a good vinaigrette dressing – especially for that wonderful appetizer, tomato with mozzarella cheese (see page 77).

RIGHT: A morning's crop of thyme, rosemary, bay, sage, tarragon, fennel and chervil. An enterprising cook would also pick the nasturtium flowers to add spice and colour to salads.

A RECIPE FOR A SPICED PICKLING VINEGAR

For the pickling of cabbage, gherkins and onions.

2 litres (3½ pts) malt vinegar
25 g (½oz) whole allspice
25g (½oz) cinnamon
25g (½oz) bruised ginger
25g (½oz) whole bay leaves
25g (½oz) white peppercorns

Layer the material to be pickled with salt in a plastic bowl for 24 to 48 hours, then rinse and drain well in a plastic colander. Place the bay, spices and vinegar in a bowl and put that into a pan of cold water. Bring the pan to the boil, then remove from the heat. Cover the pan and leave for two hours. Strain the vinegar before use. Pack the vegetables in sterile jars, cover with the vinegar and make an airtight seal to prevent the liquid evaporating.

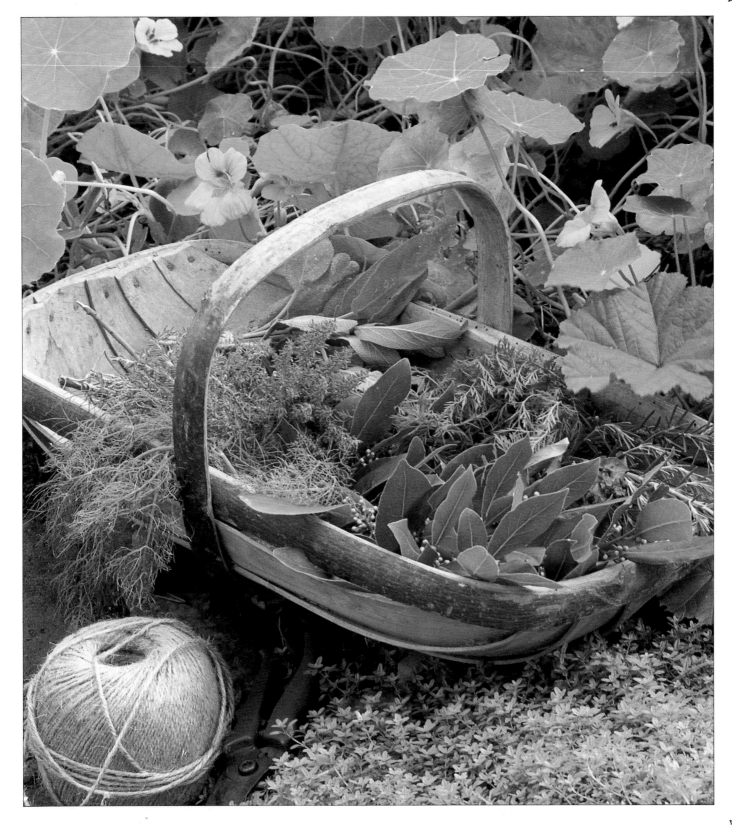

MUSTARD: A CONDIMENT AND A MEDICINE

○

'I desire your more acquaintance, good Master Mustardseed'
WILLIAM SHAKESPEARE, *A Midsummer Night's Dream*

Mustard has been used medicinally since the time of the Greek physician Hippocrates (c.460–375 BC). The Romans ate the whole seed as a spice during meals, but mustard was not milled for use at table until the eighteenth century. Today, mustard is number one in the world spice trade in terms of volume. That is perhaps a little-known fact, as most people think of spices in terms of nutmeg, mace, cinnamon, ginger and the other tropical spices and condiments.

Mustard is a temperate crop, in Britain sown in spring to produce its brilliant yellow flowers in early summer, then harvested in late summer and early autumn. It is mainly grown in East Anglia. Two different species are cultivated, *Brassica juncea* Brown Mustard and *Sinapsis alba* White Mustard. Each has a different quality to add to the blended mustard powder or creamed mustard, the brown giving pungency (and the rich yellow colour) and the white adding fire. The blending of these two characteristics can lead to many permutations and different nations have definite preferences; for example, the French use mustards creamed with vinegar and incorporate whole or partly cracked seeds, while the Americans prefer sweetened creamed mustards with a less fiery aftertaste to them.

In France the centre of the mustard trade is Dijon where a huge range is produced for blending with herb butters, and to use with poultry, egg and fish dishes, rather than the more traditional British mustard range used mainly with beef and ham.

The action of mustard as a condiment is due to three qualities. These are its ability to stimulate appetite and salivation and so hasten the first stage of digestion, its ability to break down indigestible fats and meat fibres, and its ability to stimulate digestive juices to complete the digestive process. Many people find the taste itself adds to their enjoyment, so aiding good digestion!

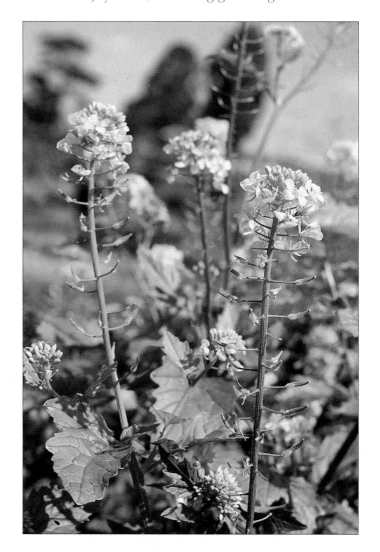

The seed of Sinapsis alba *White Mustard gives the fiery note in mustard powder preferred by the British.*

Medicinal mustard

Mustard contains an essential oil (allyl isothio-cyanate) which, when applied to the outside of the body, increases the circulation and so helps the elimination of poisons. This makes it of great value in treating a number of complaints, from a simple chill to rheumatism. Externally, mustard is often applied as a poultice or pack (for example, to ease bronchitis, neuralgia or toothache) but it is also available as an ointment. Mustard ointment has long been marketed in Britain and is recommended to ease the pain of unbroken chilblains. Two or three tablespoons of mustard powder can be used in the bath to ease chills, relax tired muscles and promote sleep. Aching feet can also benefit from a foot bath (one tablespoon) and I have found this very beneficial when I have been chilled.

Some hints for using mustard in cooking

If you are using dry mustard powder always cream it in cold water and let it stand for ten minutes before use. Make fresh for each meal.

Use dry mustard to rub over frozen joints of meat as a tenderizer before cooking.

Tenderize and flavour bacon by adding dry mustard to the frying pan before cooking.

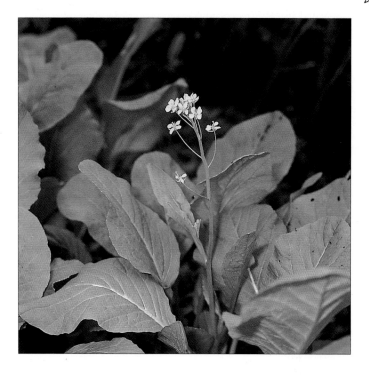

The seed of Brassica juncea *Brown Mustard gives pungency and colour to prepared mustards.*

TRADITIONAL WELSH RAREBIT

200g (½ lb) mild Cheddar cheese
1 tablespoon butter
½ teaspoon black pepper
¼ teaspoon salt
1 tablespoon milk
2 or 3 tablespoons beer
1 teaspoon made mustard

Dice the cheese. Melt the butter, and add the pepper, salt and milk to it, stirring continuously. Turn in the cheese and continue stirring until creamy and then add the beer. Continue stirring and add the mustard. Cook for a few minutes and then serve on hot toast.

A SEED MUSTARD SAUCE

For serving with rabbit or chicken

1 shallot
1 teaspoon unsalted butter
4 tablespoons dry white wine
4 tablespoons chicken stock
1 tablespoon whipping cream
¾ teaspoon Dijon mustard
1 sprig young French tarragon
1 level tablespoon seed mustard
20g (¾oz) unsalted butter
A little lemon juice, salt and pepper

Lightly sauté the chopped, peeled shallot in the teaspoon of butter. Add the wine and allow briefly to boil. Add the chicken stock and simmer to reduce by half. Allow to cool slightly, stir in the cream, Dijon mustard, seed mustard, tarragon and the rest of the butter. Season with salt, pepper and lemon juice to your preferred taste.

DESIGNING WITH COLOUR

○

The pleasure given by colour is one of the blessings that comes with the sense of sight. This is as true of designing with colourful plants as it is in art and perhaps it is no coincidence that many of the ideas about plant colour groupings come via gardeners trained in art.

Learning from example

In the nineteenth century the English painter J.M.W. Turner used colour in his work to portray light and atmosphere, banishing the conventional use of greyish foregrounds and green mid-distance pigments in favour of reds in the foreground, yellow in mid-distance and white or blue in far distance. Gertrude Jekyll, the great Victorian gardener, would certainly have known of Turner's lectures at the Royal Academy in London and some of his influence is noticeable in her border designs. Through her book *Colour in the Flower Garden* (1908) has come a direct line of influence to some of the finest of English gardens – Hestercombe and Tintinhull in Somerset, Sissinghurst in Kent, Hidcote Manor in Gloucestershire and Great Dixter in Sussex among others. The rose garden of Dumbarton Oaks, near Washington DC, shows the influence of her ideas and her theories are also popular in private gardens in New Zealand. You can gain many ideas from visiting these gardens and you may find that your ideas on colour evolve, even from the belief that no colours clash in nature.

People vary greatly in their colour preferences. We all have different psychological, emotional and physical responses to colour, and everyone's 'eye' is different. The basic principles of the artist's 'colour wheel', however, and the theories that

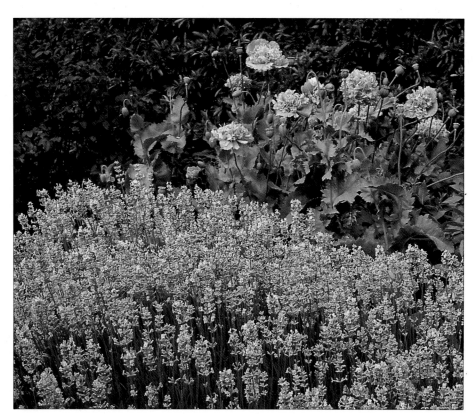

LEFT: *Pink flowers combine particularly well with grey foliage and it is surprising how often nature has contrived this in the same plant, as in the double-flowered form of the opium poppy.*
RIGHT: *The orange lilies provide a warm colour reinforced by the yellow* Hemerocallis *in front and the red* Tropaeolum speciosum.

underlie it can help you plan how colours can be grouped, mixed or matched for the most pleasing effect in your garden.

The colour wheel

In art terms there are three primary colours: red, yellow and blue. When any two of these are mixed in paint they produce the secondary colours of orange (from red and yellow), violet (from red and blue) and green (from blue and yellow). When placed next to each other in a circle the result is a 'wheel' of six basic colours.

Three adjacent colours on the wheel, sharing a common pigment, are termed 'harmonies', while colours that do not share pigments are called 'contrasts'. In the garden, as in colour design generally, it is conventionally thought best not to combine harmonies with contrasts.

Colours that are diagonally opposite on the colour wheel are called 'complementary' colours and when placed next to each other seem to intensify the depth of the other. Thus a blue flower will appear far more blue when planted next to an orange or yellow one or when seen immediately after it, such as a border of blue flowers leading into a border of yellows.

The American psychologist Bivven did some research in the 1960s that showed that most people respond most positively to closely harmonious or complementary colours or to strong contrasting colours.

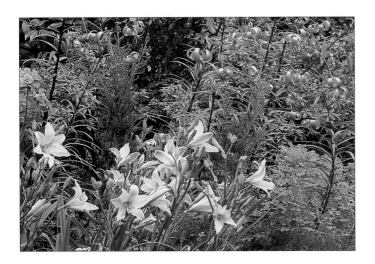

Theory in practice

Designers also speak of the 'temperature' of a colour. Reds and oranges are considered to be warm colours, while blues are thought to be cool. In general, warm colours seem to advance towards the eye; for example, red is a bright, hot colour that is immediately noticeable in a flower border. Cooler colours seem to recede from the eye, mirroring the effect of looking into the distance at the horizon. Thus blue flowers can add an impression of perspective and depth to a flower border, increasing the feeling of space.

In art the tone of a colour can be modified by the addition of varying amounts of black or white paint. This theory can also be used in the garden, where the colours of flowers can be affected by being placed near to white flowers or to grey-leaved plants. For example, a phlox of a particularly vivid magenta can be toned down and look far more attractive when planted behind the grey *Stachys byzantina*.

Remember that climate can affect your appreciation of colour. It is easier to design with strong colours in bright subtropical light and with softer ones in the more subdued light of temperate climates. Light also changes throughout the day. Thus it is easier to design gardens of warm harmonious colours for enjoyment close to sunrise or sunset. Gardens that feature mainly blue flowers appear at their best in the light of noon.

Colours can also vary according to the texture of the leaf or petal. A heavily textured leaf has areas of shadow and can appear to look darker. It will also look different when wet; try seeing a garden's colours afresh when the rain stops and the sun comes out!

Be conscious of nature's seasonal palettes. For example, pink is rare in late summer, yellow is commonest in spring and late summer whereas true blues and pale yellows are rare altogether.

Persevere to become as skilled at using colours as the flower breeders are in producing it. Design to please yourself and do not be afraid to use colours that have pleasant memories of people or places for you alone. That in itself is therapeutic.

COLOUR AND MOOD

○

In the past few decades much attention has been paid by interior designers to the way that colour in the home can affect mood and express personality. Since Penelope Hobhouse made a radical advance on Gertrude Jekyll's theories of colour in the garden in her book *Colour in Your Garden* (1985) there has been a revival of interest in colour associations between plants as outdoor design features.

However, the concept of colour as 'healing' – in the sense of being designed to ameliorate mood – is rarely mentioned. Yet this is the logical extension of the use of colour in interior design, especially with the modern perception of town or courtyard gardens as being 'outdoor rooms' and an extension of living space. It is quite possible to design both foliage and flower colour in your garden to create certain desired effects to match or to change your mood. Here are some suggestions, colour by colour, for you to consider, followed on pages 86–91 by detailed plant lists for particular border colour groupings.

Red

Red is said to be the first colour perceived by infants and the first colour to be named in a developing language. It has physical effects on us (perhaps because of its association with blood), quickening the heart rate and stimulating the body to produce adrenalin. It is a dominant colour that advances visually. This can tire both the eye and mind and traditionally it has been difficult to place in the garden. In nature, red is also a warning colour and it may be that we subconsciously recognize this.

On the other hand, in strong light (such as that of the Mediterranean) red can be a joyful colour and when blended with other rich colours and backgrounds, such as mellow stone, it can produce a warming psychological response.

Red is best used to produce glorious effects in the strong light of late summer. It is a comparatively rare colour in the palette of early summer-flowering species. The complementary colour to red is mid-green, so the foliage of non-purple leaved varieties increases the intensity of red, as does an adjacent lawn. Some people find the blue-reds emotionally 'colder' than the yellow-reds. Excellent 'red borders' can be seen at Hidcote Manor in Gloucestershire and red is often used to startling effect in some of Tuscany's most famous gardens, including the Villa Gamberaia outside Florence.

Pink

Many people find pink a warm, inviting colour. It is one that harmonizes with many others, producing a soft, restful effect, particularly when teamed with grey-leaved plants. Pink also retains its colour well into the evening. Be careful, however, to choose soft pinks. There are many strident pinks among modern hybrids that are anything but restful to the eye.

Green

Green appears restful in all its variations; it is a neutral colour, containing both warm yellow and cool blue. It neither advances nor recedes visually and thus does not tire the eye. Gardens designed entirely around the various greens of foliage can be extremely subtle and peaceful. Foliage is also a constant throughout the growing season where floral effects can be temporary and sometimes look more contrived, so a green garden is recommended for long-lasting effect.

Yellow

Yellow has had some negative associations in religious art, as the colour of betrayal and persecution; and it is often associated with ill health, ill luck, cowardice and stupidity in Western folklore. Pale, sulphur yellows are actually quite rare in garden plants whereas gold – traditionally associated with kingship, wisdom and riches – is profuse, particularly in spring and late summer. Rich

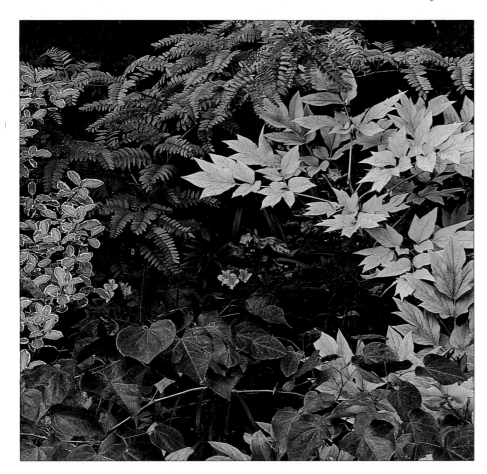

People who design gardens around foliage rather than flower find that not all leaves are green and green itself is a varied colour. Foliage also changes at different stages of the plant's life, as in the bronzed young fronds of the fern (top), and with the splendours of autumn colour.

yellow is the colour of sunshine and is cheering. Overall, yellow is one of the commonest colours in flowers and, because it is very reflective, it is often planted in gardens designed for evening use. It cheers the spirit and is easily seen in poor light. Yellow needs good foliage accompaniment to enrich its effect.

Orange

Orange is a challenge in the garden, but it can be extraordinarily warm and rich (and produce a corresponding mood) when teamed with purple or bronze-leaved plants and backed by deep greens such as yew hedges.

Blue

Blue is usually thought of as the colour of reverie and of dreams, perhaps because of its links with the sky and sea. It is a sedating colour that calms the mind and suggests the infinite. However, it can veer off into sadness and depression ('singing the blues') if not lifted by complementary colours. In the garden it can be used to increase the sense of space of those who feel cramped; it recedes from the eye visually, lengthening perspective and giving spatial depth.

True blues are quite rare in plants and usually verge towards violet or purple. Totally blue borders are, to my mind, visually unalluring and quite cold in their effect. Mid-blues mixed with soft pinks, white and silver foliage, however, can give a pretty, but restful, effect. Violet blues are best mixed with yellows to increase visual interest. Pale blues can be charming in a very informal setting – such as the glorious effect of the bluebells at the Royal Botanic Gardens, Kew, England, where they are mixed with the lime green of *Smyrnium perfoliatum.*

A HARMONY OF WARM COLOURS

○

The use of harmonious colour in the 'hot' part of the colour wheel – the reds and oranges – can be used in a garden to produce a warm response in the observer. This is particularly true if this type of colour scheme is sited as a surprise. A border chanced upon when turning a corner, a 'garden within a garden', or a grouping of plants in a separate courtyard, for example, will create a strong emotional effect.

Suggestions for planting

You are only likely to be able to design a full border of reds and oranges at certain times of the year because there are comparatively few red-flowering perennials that flower in early summer. The 'hottest' borders come into their own from mid summer onwards when a plethora of strong colours are available, perhaps suggestive of the maturing year and the move towards the rich colours of autumn after the fresher colours of spring. All the American members of the daisy family – *Helenium*, *Rudbeckia*, *Solidago* to name but a few – come into their own, and many writers have suggested that the best way of toning this exuberant outburst is to plant with copper or purple-leaved plants. An example of where such planting is done well is in the South Cottage Garden at Sissinghurst Castle in Kent, England. Planting orange-flowered perennials where the evening sun will catch them (particularly if backed by a wall of warm-coloured stone) will also enrich the observer's eye.

Red borders are at their best in mid to late summer. If you feel really daring, try a border of red and purple-leaved plants for late-summer effect. The best materials to use are red-flowered herbaceous plants and purple-leaved deciduous shrubs. Species to choose from include *Cotinus coggygria* 'Notcutt's Purple', *Prunus × cistena*, *Dahlia* 'Bishop of Llandaff', *Cosmos atrosanguineus*, *Berberis thunbergii* 'Atropurpurea' and, in light shade, *Acer palmatum* 'Atropurpureum'. Plant these so that the lengthening rays of the sun in the afternoon and evening catch the purple foliage from behind and enliven it. However, beware of reds that contain some blue in their pigment. Keep these separate from the hot-colour groupings I have suggested in flame, orange, copper and bronze. They are all colour combinations that I have noticed over the past ten years and noted as very successful. Most horticultural colour theorists recommend that these hot colours that have yellow in their make-up, do not tone well with hot colours that contain blue, such as the magentas, mauves and soft crimsons. I would agree – but it is important for you to try for yourself.

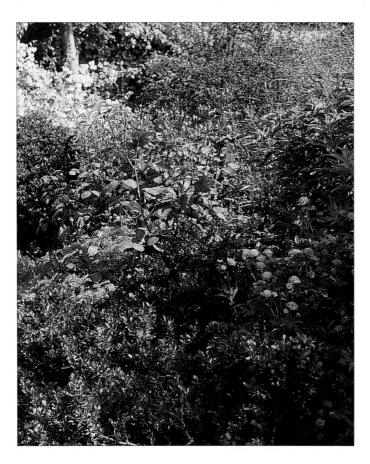

Red flowers combine harmoniously with purple leaves.

WARM COLOUR BORDERS

Yellow, flame and orange flowers can be developed and enriched by close proximity to shrubs with copper or bronze foliage. You can mix and match these suggested groupings provided you can supply the right aspect and soil conditions for them. Grade the plants in height according to the guides given so that no plant swamps or obscures its neighbours but is given full room to develop properly.

HOT COLOUR GROUPINGS IN FLAME, ORANGE AND COPPER/BRONZE

Yellow/Flame/Orange	Copper/Bronze (Foliage)	Comment
Geum chiloense 'Mrs Bradshaw' 30 × 30cm (12 × 12in) *Geum* 'Borisii' 60 × 45cm (2 × 1½ft) *Ranunculus acris* 'Flore Pleno' 75 × 45cm (2½ × 1½ft) *Hemerocallis dumortierii* 60 × 45cm (2 × 1½ft)	*Rheum palmatum* 'Atrosanguineum' 1.5 × 1.5m (5 × 5ft) and *Crocosmia* 'Solfatare' 75 × 25cm (30 × 10in)	A lovely, rich grouping for the mid border.
Inula magnifica 1.8 × 1m (6 × 3ft) Red or yellow *Hemerocallis* 60–90 × 45cm (2–3 × 1½ft)	*Ligularia dentata* 'Desdemona' or 'Othello' or 'Moorblut' 1.5 × 1m (5 × 3ft)	Best in moist soil.
Potentilla 'Gibson's Scarlet' 30 × 60cm (1 × 2ft) *Achillea filipendulina* 'Gold Plate' 1.5–2.5 × 1.8–2.5m (5–8 × 6–8ft)	*Dahlia* 'Bishop of Llandaff' 1–1.5 × 1m (3–5 × 3ft) or purple-leaved Cannas such as 'Egandale' and 'Wyoming' 1–1.5 × 0.45m (3–5 × 1½ft)	Must have full sun.
Euphorbia griffithii 'Fireglow' 75 × 60cm (2.5 × 2ft) *Azalea* 'Knaphill hybrids' 1.5–2.5 × 1.8–2.5m (5–8 × 6–8ft)	*Corylus maxima* 'Purpurea' 5.5 × 5.5m (18 × 18ft)	Acid soil needed.
Calendula officinalis 30 × 30cm (12 × 12in) *Lilium* 'Enchantment' or *Lilium bulbiferum* var. *croceum* or *Lilium* × *hollandicum* 0.6–1.2m × 10cm (2–4 × 4ft)	*Prunus* × *cistena* 1.8 × 1.8m (6 × 6ft)	The *Prunus* could form a backing hedge.
Primula bulleyana, *P. chungensis*, *P. aurantiaca* 60–75 × 45cm (2–2½ × 1½ft)	*Rheum palmatum* 'Atrosanguineum' 1.5 × 1.5m (5 × 5ft) *Lobelia cardinalis* 90 × 30cm (3 × 1ft) *Rodgersia aesculifolia* 1.8 × 0.75m (6 × 2½ft)	Must have moist soil.
Inula 'Golden Beauty' 1.2 × 1m (4 × 3ft) *Helenium* cultivars 0.6–1.5 × 0.45m (2–5 × 1½ft)	*Phormium tenax* 'Purpureum' 2 × 1.2m (7 × 4ft) *Salvia officinalis* 'Purpurascens' (in front) 0.6 × 1.5m (2 × 5ft)	Full sun needed.

COMPLEMENTARY BLUES AND YELLOWS

Colours appear what they are not, according to the ground which surrounds them,' wrote Leonardo da Vinci, an idea taken up by the French Impressionist painters in the 1880s. Through her interest in both painting and gardens, Gertrude Jekyll took the nineteenth-century preoccupation with colour theory into garden design, particularly with regard to the use of complementary colours.

One of the effects of pairs of complementary colours such as blue and orange, violet and yellow, and red and green, is that each colour physically induces an after-image of its partner in the eye, even when it is closed. This simple fact can be exploited by garden designers to intensify colour by preparing the eye in advance. For example, an area of gold foliage preceding a block of violet-blue planting will enhance that planting by its after-image effect. The eye yearns for the colour's complement and then is satisfied by it.

As Gertrude Jekyll wrote in *Colour in the Flower Garden* (1908), 'Now the eye has again become saturated, and has therefore, by the law of complementary colour, acquired a strong appetite for the greys and purples. These therefore assume an appearance of brilliancy that they would not have had without the preparation provided by their recently received complementary colour.'

Suggestions for planting

One way of using complementary colours is to design single-colour gardens that lead into one another but are physically separated by hedges. Thus a yellow garden would be followed by a blue garden, or vice versa. The eye is then successively prepared and refreshed as the observer moves around the garden.

Yellow tulips and blue myosotis combine effectively for a spring bedding display, the blue enriching the yellow to the eye.

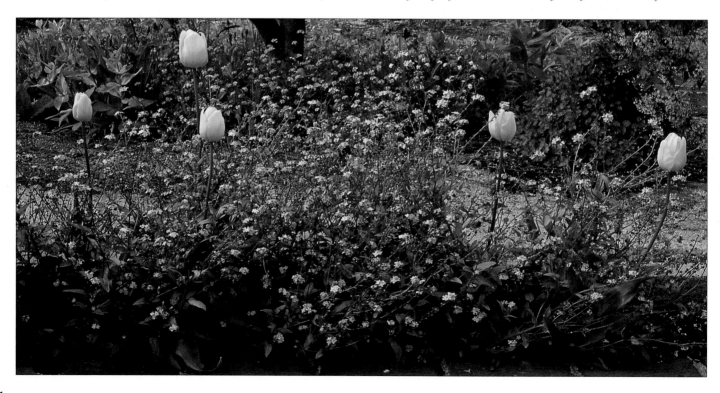

In a border where you wish to use blue and yellow try grading the blues from one end of the border to the other, using yellows as groupings within this to produce a rich and unified visual effect. Arrange the various tones of blue carefully, say with the pale and mid-blues interspersed with the gold or orange-yellows and the violet-blues with the paler yellows. This is quite a feat of planting design and is complicated by the fact that blues will often be deeper in alkaline soils.

You will have to work hard to find good sulphur-yellows: *Potentilla fruticosa* 'Primrose Beauty' and *Potentilla recta sulphurea* are good ones, as is the lovely *Achillea* 'Moonshine', not seen as often as its brassier companion *Achillea filipendulina* 'Gold Plate'. I would also avoid using gold-foliaged plants

BLUE AND YELLOW BORDERS

Blue and yellow visually enrich each other as colours by the law of complementary colour, and seem particularly fresh in spring displays of bulbs and herbaceous plants. See page 90 for suggestions for summer planting and for using autumn leaf colour and autumn-flowering bulbs in the blue and yellow ranges.

BLUE AND YELLOW GROUPINGS FOR SPRING

Blue	Yellow	Comment
Hyacinthoides non-scripta 30 × 15cm (12 × 6in)	*Rhododendron luteum* 3 × 3m (10 × 10ft)	For a woodland garden on acid soil.
Crocus sieberi or *C. tomasinianus* 6 × 5cm (2½ × 2in)	*Cornus mas* 3 × 3m (10 × 10ft)	Plant the *Cornus* as a lawn specimen underplanted with the *Crocus*.
Scilla sibirica or *Anemone apennina* (blue form) 15–20 × 10cm (6–8 × 4in)	*Forsythia suspensa* 3 × 2.5m (10 × 8ft)	Plant the bulbs in drifts under the *Forsythia*.
Ceanothus impressus 1.5 × 1.8m (5 × 6ft)	*Tulip* 'Mrs Moon' 45 × 18cm (18 × 6in) *Coronilla glauca* 3 × 2.5m (10 × 8ft) *Rosa* 'Helen Knight' 3 × 2m (10 × 7ft)	For a warm border. Train the rose on a wall behind.
Brunnera macrophylla or *Omphalodes cappodocica* 30–45 × 30–45cm (12–18 × 12–18in)	*Doronicum austriacum* 60 × 30cm (2 × 1ft)	For good, moist soil.
Myosotis sylvatica 15–40 × 15cm (6–16 × 6in)	*Millium effusum* 'Aureum' 45 × 30cm (18 × 12in)	Both of these will seed about.
Omphalodes cappodocica 30–45 × 30–45cm (12–18 × 12–18in)	*Euphorbia polychroma* 45 × 45cm (18 × 18in)	Use close to the front of a border.
Meconopsis betonicifolia or *M. grandis* 90 × 45cm (3ft × 18in)	*Primula helodoxa* or *P. florindae* 90 × 45cm (3ft × 18in)	Late spring. For acid soil.

BLUE AND YELLOW GROUPINGS FOR SUMMER

Blue	Yellow	Comment
Geranium sylvaticum 'Mayflower' 75 × 60cm (2.5 × 2ft)	*Cytisus × praecox* 1.8 × 1.8m (6 × 6ft)	Must have full sun.
Geranium 'Johnson's Blue' and blue *Iris sibirica* cultivars both 90 × 60cm (3 × 2ft)	*Rosa* 'Golden Wings' 1.8 × 1.5m (6 × 5ft) *Rosa* 'Frühlingsgold' 2 × 2m (7 × 7ft)	Must have full sun.
Campanula lactiflora 1 × 0.6cm (3 × 2ft)	*Lilium × testaceum* 1.5 × 0.3m (5 × 1ft)	Both need rich, moist soil.
Lobelia syphilitica 1 × 0.3m (3 × 1ft)	*Primula florindae* 1 × 0.6m (3 × 2ft)	Needs moist soil or bog.
Lavandula spica 1 × 1m (3 × 3ft)	*Potentilla* 'Primrose Beauty' 1 × 1m (3 × 3ft)	This makes a good mixed low hedge in sun and poorish soil.
Salvia farinacea 'Victoria' or *S. haematodes* 'Indigo' 45 × 30cm (18 × 12in)	*Alchemilla mollis* 30 × 60cm (12 × 24in)	As used at Hidcote Manor, Gloucestershire, England.
Salvia guaranitica 1.5 × 0.6m (5 × 2ft)	*Hypericum* 'Rowallane' 2 × 2m (7 × 7ft)	As used at Knighthayes Court, Devon, England. Warm gardens only.
Stokesia laevis 45 × 45cm (18 × 18in)	*Achillea* 'Moonshine' 60 × 45cm (2 × 1.5ft)	A soft colour combination.
Clematis 'Xerxes' 2.5–3.5 × 3m (8–10 × 10ft) *Campanula carpatica* or *C. portenschlagiana* 15 × 90cm (6in × 3ft)	*Rosa* 'Golden Wings' 1.8 × 1.5cm (6 × 5ft)	Clematis on wall backing the rose. The campanula is used as an edging.
Thalictrum speciosissimum (purple) 1.5 × 1m (5 × 3ft) and *Lythrum salicaria* (purple) 1.2 × 0.6m (4 × 2ft)	*Lysimachia vulgaris* 90 × 60cm (3 × 2ft)	For damp soil.

BLUE AND YELLOW GROUPINGS FOR AUTUMN

Blue	Yellow	Comment
Autumn-flowering crocus, for example *C. speciosus* *C. banaticus* or *C. laevigatus fontenayi* all 12 × 9cm (5 × 3in)	*Morus alba* 4.5 × 4.5m (15 × 15ft)	Crocus form a blue underplanting for the Mulberry's yellow autumn leaf colour.
Ceratostigma plumbaginoides 1 × 1m (3 × 3ft)	*Arundinaria viridistriata* (Golden Bamboo) 1.2 × 1m (4 × 3ft) backed by *Mahonia undulata* 2.5 × 1.5m (6 × 5ft)	*Ceratostigma* is used as an edging.

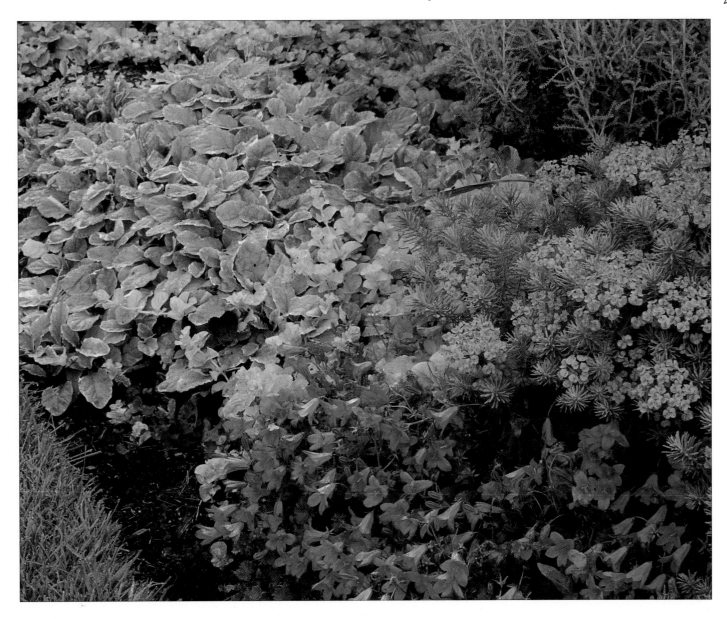

except for spring borders, because the colour often fades as the sun becomes higher in the sky towards mid summer and the foliage may burn in a border fully exposed to the sunshine that most border plants require. Plan your border against a good green hedge as a background or against an orangey brick wall – blues and yellows look far less stunning against a fence.

Use the table to design groups within your border – for spring, for summer or for autumn effect. Some of the suggested spring groupings have

The intense blue of Campanula portenschlagiana *is deepened by proximity to the yellow foliage of Creeping Jenny* Lysimachia nummularia *'Aurea'.*

been used at the Royal Botanic Gardens, Kew, where an adventurous use of colour with perennial plants has been developed since the mid-1960s. Other gardens where colour effects are well used include Villandry in the French Loire Valley, Versailles outside Paris and the Botanic Gardens in Auckland, New Zealand.

STRUCTURE AND SHAPE

People can obtain great visual pleasure from a well-structured garden, both in its planting and its overall design. Whatever your taste in garden design and style, a plan that satisfies the eye can infuse a strong sense of psychological well-being, setting important 'boundaries'. Several good design partnerships in this century have evolved with one partner designing the 'hard' constructional, non-living elements of the garden and the other the 'soft' element of the planting.

A pleasing outlook

Landscape architects and garden designers frequently talk of the 'bones' of a garden, by which they mean its built landscape features such as walls, terraces, paths, pergolas and other elements that define the basic plan and provide a framework for the plants.

Structure can also be provided by hedges, either tall ones that give shelter and form a backdrop or dwarf hedges, perhaps of box or santolina, that are traditionally used in herb and knot gardens. Long avenues that end in a statue or sculpture can give distinct pleasure when first glimpsed.

Similar visual satisfaction can be gained from a deliberately framed view through a gate, a 'window' in a wall, an arch or a hole in a hedge.

Containers of various kinds, such as urns and terracotta pots, can be used as an 'end stop' to a flowing border or at the intersection of paths. Strong colour can sometimes prove very effective in the plants chosen for these, acting almost like punctuation in the overall design.

The sense of internal space within a garden can be made more diverse by changes in level. Terracing is used in most Italian Renaissance gardens, and sunken gardens were common in Edwardian England, one being the fine Lutyens/Jekyll designed garden at Hestercombe in Somerset. Dumbarton Oaks outside Washington DC is similarly planned. Walled sunken gardens often act as effective suntraps and thus give additional enjoyment, as well as protection to plants.

BELOW LEFT: Plants can be sculptures in their own right, as with the water-loving Gunnera manicata.
BELOW: Hard structures in the garden such as the wall with a moongate frame views and divide the internal space.

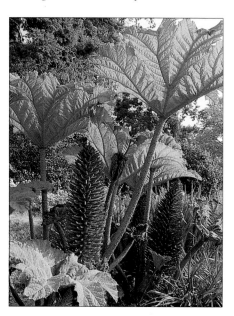

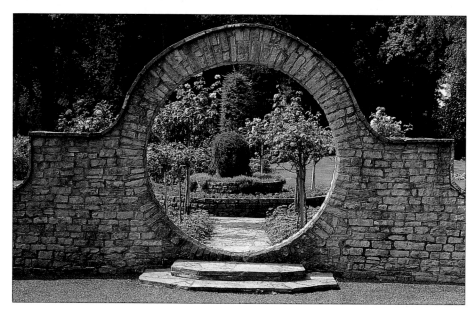

PLANT OUTLINES

Botanical name/Common name	Maximum height and spread	Comment
Acanthus species	1.2 × 1m (4 × 3ft)	For full sun. Perennial. Sp
Bergenia cordifolia and cultivars	30 × 45cm (12 × 18in)	Any soil, shade. Perennial. H
Betula pendula 'Dalecarlica' or 'Youngii'	11 × 4.5m (36 × 15ft)	Dainty trees. S
Crocosmia species and varieties	60–75 × 25cm (24–30 × 10in)	For full sun. Perennial. Sp
Eriobotrya japonica Loquat	5.5 × 4.5m (18 × 15ft)	Shrub for warm gardens. H
Fatsia japonica	2 × 2m (7 × 7ft)	Makes a good specimen shrub. H
Ferns – all types	Variable	Need semi-shade. Perennial. S
Grasses – all types	Variable	Mostly need full sun. Perennial. S
Gunnera manicata	3 × 3.5m (10 × 12ft)	For bog gardens. Perennial. H
Hosta, most varieties	up to 45 × 45cm (18 × 18in)	Moist soil, shade. Perennial. H
Indigofera species	1.8 × 1.5m (6 × 5ft)	Good on dry soil. Shrub. S
Iris spuria and *I. sibirica* cultivars	1–1.2 × 0.6m (3–4 × 2ft)	For full sun. Perennial. Sp
Paulownia species Foxglove Trees	9 × 9m (30 × 30ft)	For warm gardens. H
Phormium tenax and *P. colensoi* cultivars New Zealand Flax	species to 3 × 1.5m (10 × 5ft)	Dwarf cultivars available. Perennial. Sp
Tamarix species	4.5 × 4.5m (15 × 15ft)	Need full sun. Shrub. S
Yucca species	0.6–3 × 1.2m (2–10 × 4ft)	Very architectural shrubs. Sp.
Zantedeschia aethiopica	90 × 60cm (3 × 2ft)	For moist or wet soils. Perennial. H

KEY: H hard outline   S soft outline   Sp spiky leaved

Shapes of plants

The shapes of plants themselves are an important part of good garden design. This is sometimes called 'form' in garden design; that is, the overall combination of spiky, rounded, conical and feathery outlines that give three-dimensional shape to a planting. You can choose from a wide variety of trees, shrubs and perennials that can be combined and contrasted to give a pleasing balance of soft, hard-edged and spiky plants.

Some species fulfil several patterns in that they have large hard-edged leaves and delicate masses of feathery flowers; for example, *Crambe cordifolia* and *Crambe maritima*. Here the fourth dimension in garden design is introduced, that of time. The effect a plant gives may well depend on its growth stage at a particular time of year. For example, the *Crambe* has clearly defined edges in spring but is soft when covered with profuse panicles of flowers in early summer. Many conifers look hard in outline except in early spring as their soft new growth appears

Some unusually shaped plants can be used almost as sculptures in the garden. The Monkey Puzzle *Araucaria araucana* is a good candidate for this sort of treatment as are some of the *Phormium* species. Other architectural plants are palms and agaves. Plants with strong leaves are best placed against a hard landscaped background for their form to be enjoyed.

THE SPECIAL EFFECT OF A WHITE GARDEN

○

The popularity of gardens with white or cream flowers counterpointed against green foliage has received an enormous boost from the success of Vita Sackville-West's white garden at Sissinghurst Castle in Kent, internationally known as one of Britain's finest gardens. Other white gardens can be seen at Hidcote Manor in Gloucestershire and Newby Hall in Yorkshire.

White at night

White gardens are particularly appreciated in the summer for evening use by those who are out at work all day. White becomes almost luminous at night and generates an ethereal quality at dusk just when other colours are fading to shadows. The texture of petals, whether shiny or matt, and the relative boldness or airiness of white flower-heads is also more noticeable in the twilight.

A white garden in the evening is also frequently a fragrant garden as so many white-flowered plants exude scent at night in the competition to attract night-flying moths for pollination.

White also has its own psychological associations. Traditionally, in Christian religious art white flowers reflect purity, innocence and the infinite and eternal, and a pot of Madonna lilies *Lilium candidum* on the terrace is sure to strike a chord for many people.

City dwellers may find the cleanliness of white refreshing after a day of urban pollution.

Designing with white

White reflects and contains all other colours and thus can be deeply calming; it does not challenge (which is why it is so useful in interior design) and its stillness can be used effectively in court-yards or gardens planned as 'outdoor rooms'.

White is also a relief from stronger colour and can lead to a quiet appreciation of subtlety in its effect against green and grey, and indeed in the different variations of white itself. (No wonder that the Inuit Eskimos have seventeen different words to describe whiteness!)

A well-designed white garden concentrates on designing for flowers at the time of year when evenings are longest and the special quality of white at night can best be appreciated. Use strongly grouped plants with bold flower shapes to waymark the paths and boundaries of the garden and site outdoor lighting in appropriate places to highlight the effect.

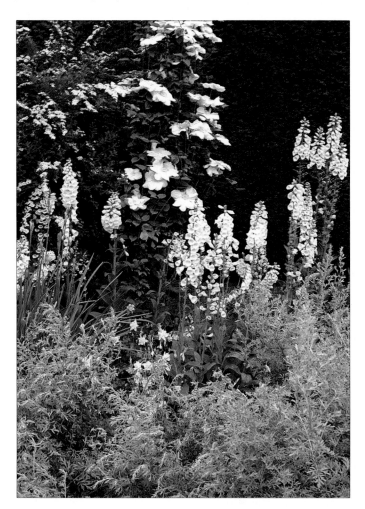

White flowers mix well with green and grey foliage.

A WHITE PLANTING TO BE ENJOYED IN EARLY SUMMER

Start by plotting the structure: trees and most significant shrubs. Then fill in with perennials in groups of three or five. Plant bulbs between and among them.

Use climbers on tripods for vertical accent if your area does not include walls. Finally, plant annuals in pots, tubs or in any gaps in front of your composition.

Botanical name	Maximum height and spread	Comment
TREES		
Halesia caroliniana	7.5 × 7.5m (25 × 25ft)	Best tree for the average-sized garden.
Styrax japonica	6 × 6m (20 × 20ft)	Best tree for the small-sized garden.
PERENNIALS		
Campanula alliariifolia 'Ivory Bells'	60 × 45cm (2 × 1½ft)	Very elegant pendant flowers.
Crambe cordifolia	1.8 × 1.2m (6 × 4ft)	Creates a haze of white flowers.
Dianthus 'Mrs Sinkins'	30 × 30–45cm (12 × 12–18in)	For a dry, sunny spot. Good on chalk soils.
Dicentra eximia 'Alba'	30–45 × 30cm (12–18 × 12in)	Needs moisture.
Digitalis purpurea – white strains	1.2 × 0.3m (4 × 1ft)	Best in semi-shade.
Hesperis matronalis	1 × 0.6m (3 × 2ft)	Lovely at night when it is also scented.
Papaver orientale 'Black and White'	60 × 60cm (2 × 2ft)	Full sun needed.
Zantedeschia aethiopica	90 × 60cm (3 × 2ft)	Needs moist soil and light shade.
SHRUBS		
Carpentaria californica	1.8 × 1.8m (6 × 6ft)	Only for warm gardens.
Cistus laurifolius	1.8 × 1.8m (6 × 6ft)	One of the hardiest of the *Cistus*.
Convolvulus cneorum	1 × 1m (3 × 3ft)	Must have full sun.
Cornus kousa 'Chinensis'	4 × 3m (13 × 10ft)	Needs acid soil.
Philadelphus species hybrids and cultivars	up to 3 × 2.5m (10 × 8ft)	Lovely, but short flowering season.
Pittosporum tobira	4.5 × 3.5m (15 × 12ft)	Only for very warm gardens.
Rosa 'Iceberg'	1–1.2 × 1m (3–4 × 3ft)	May need spraying against mildew.
Syringa 'Madame Lemoine'	3.5 × 3m (12 × 10ft)	Lovely, but short flowering season.
Viburnum plicatum 'Lanarth'	3 × 3m (10 × 10ft)	Best in moist soil and light shade.
BULBS		
Camassia leichtlinii (white form)	1.2 × 0.3m (4 × 1ft)	Needs a warm position.
Convallaria majalis	20 × 30cm (8 × 12in)	Spreads if it is happy.
Lilium regale	1.2 × 0.3m (4 × 1ft)	One of the best lilies for style and scent.
ANNUALS		
Argemone grandiflora	90 × 30cm (3 × 1ft)	Delicate flowers.
Lavatera 'Mont Blanc'	60 × 30cm (2 × 1ft)	Icy white petals.
Nicotiana alata	90 × 30cm (3 × 1ft)	Flowers open in the evening.
CLIMBERS		
Jasminum officinale	9 × 4m (30 × 15ft)	Requires training, will not self-cling.
Wisteria sinensis 'Alba'	20 × 20m (65 × 65ft)	Requires spur pruning in winter.

HEALING SOUNDS IN THE GARDEN

○

Your garden can become a refuge from the noise pollution of the urban and workaday world and the disturbance and stresses that unwanted noise produces.

From the sighing and rustling of leaves and stems in the breeze to the tinkling or rushing of water, sounds in the garden can generate and influence many different moods and feelings. Sounds, like scent, can trigger vivid memories and can bring to mind happy incidents in the past, often from childhood. These can have a psychologically healing effect, especially against depression and as an antidote to the strains of everyday pressures and uncertainties.

Wind and water

Refreshing sounds can be produced by the movement of the wind through trees and shrubs, and there are many species you can plant for this purpose (see table). Bamboos and grasses give gentle rustling sounds that can provide a pleasing background to more immediate sounds, as can running or falling water.

Waterfalls and fountains, producing a trickle or cascade, can be 'tuned' through careful arrangement of the height, angle and interruption of the fall of water to make 'scales' of sound, bringing an added dimension of harmony to a garden. Further ideas about the use of running water to provide refreshing sounds are given on page 99.

The sounds of insects

Choosing plants that create sounds is a start, but there are also many other species that attract sounds to them. Plants and flowers that are irresistible to insects will result in a glorious drowsy hum on a sunny summer's afternoon as the bees and others busy themselves among the blooms. You can deliberately plant to attract bees by specifically selecting species they use as sources

LEFT: Bamboos produce a constant rustling sound in the slightest breeze, but do choose a non-invasive species.
BELOW: Salix exiqua, like many willows, is often planted by water, so introducing other sounds by the wildlife it attracts.

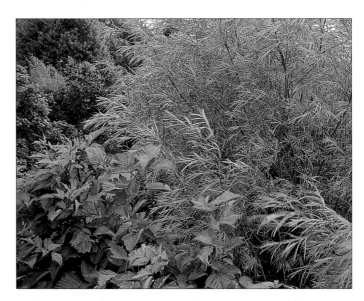

of nectar or pollen. Some of the best to plant are any of the varieties of thyme, lavender and rosemary, *Phlomis*, *Lythrum*, *Eryngium*, *Cytisus*, *Verbena* and particularly *Cistus*, which also provide scent and colour in the garden.

At the Chelsea Physic Garden, where we keep bees, large numbers have been recorded on *Rosa pimpinellifolia*, *Mirabilis jalapa*, the Fuller's Teasel *Dipsacus fullonum*, many of the paeonies and all of the Californian Lilacs (*Ceanothus* species and varieties). Further ways to attract other wildlife to the garden are suggested on page 144.

TREES, SHRUBS AND GRASSES TO PLEASE THE EAR

Botanical name	Common name	Maximum height and spread	Comment
Betula papyrifera	Paper birch	9 × 4.5m (30 × 15ft)	Where a light textured tree is wanted.
Colutea arborescens	Bladder senna	1.8 × 2.5m (6 × 8ft)	The pods rattle and rustle in the breeze.
Cordyline australis	Cabbage palm	3.5 × 2.5m (12 × 8ft)	The strap-shaped leaves rustle together.
Cornus florida	Flowering dogwood	4.5 × 4.5m (15 × 15ft)	For a woodland garden.
Eucalyptus	Gum trees	Variable but at least 9 × 4.5m (30 × 15ft)	For a sunny garden where the leaf litter can be crunched underfoot.
Ficus carica	Fig	4.5 × 3.5m (15 × 12ft)	For a warm wall.
Fraxinus ornus	Manna ash	6 × 6m (20 × 20ft)	For unrestricted space.
Magnolia grandiflora	Bull Bay magnolia	7.5 × 4.5m (20 × 15ft)	For a warm wall.
Miscanthus		1–3 × 1m (3–9 × 3ft)	Perennial grasses for small gardens.
Phormium tenax	New Zealand Flax	1.8–3 × 1.2m (6–10 × 4ft)	For warm gardens.
Phyllostachys nigra	Black Bamboo	3–6 × 6m (10–20 × 20ft)	Bamboo for unrestricted space.
Phyllostachys viridi-glaucescens		4.5–6 × 6m (15–20 × 20ft)	Bamboo for unrestricted space.
Picea breweriana	Brewer's weeping spruce	6 × 2.5m (20 × 8ft)	A charming spruce for the characteristic sound of the breeze in conifers.
Pinus bungeana	Lacebark pine	3.5 × 1.5m (12 × 5ft)	A suitable pine for the characteristic sound of the breeze in conifers.
Populus tremula	Aspen	12 × 9m (40 × 30ft)	For 'tremulous' sound.
Populus tremuloides	American Aspen	6–9 × 4.5m (20–30 × 15ft)	For 'tremulous' sound.
Sinarundinaria nitida	Bamboo	2.5–4 × 2m (8–13 × 7ft)	For gentle rustling sound.

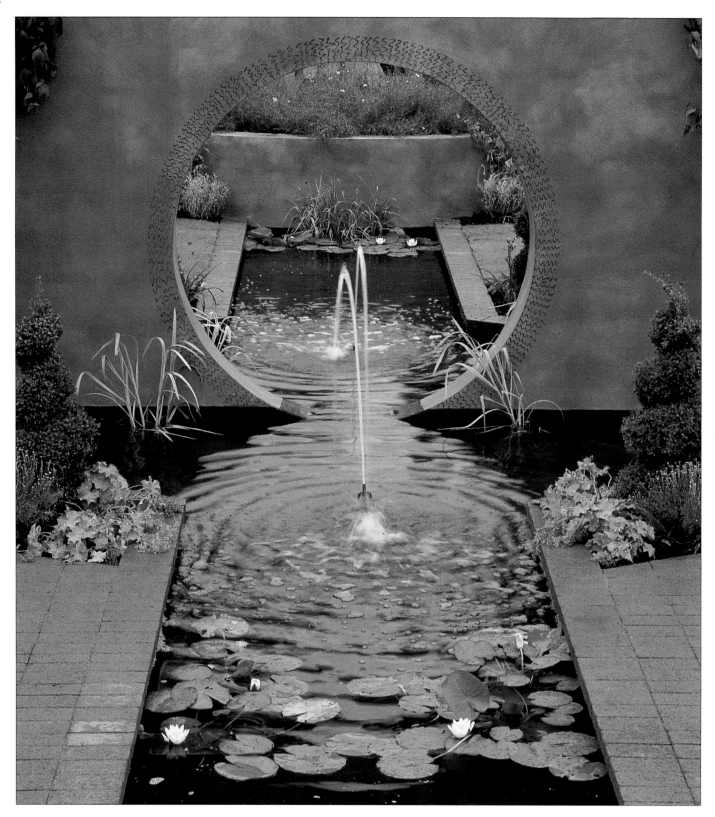

THE SOUND OF RUNNING WATER

Moving water is a wonderfully refreshing feature in a garden, cooling the air and delighting the ear. It exerts a fascination of its own, quite different from the effect of tranquil sheets of water.

For centuries the design of water gardens with large cascades and fountains was the preserve of the rich for it relied on expensive substantial reservoirs and pumphouses. Today, using the range of submersible pumps that are available, anyone can enjoy a modest fountain or moving-water feature in their garden. If it is sited near the house, patio or a conservatory the sound is especially appreciated. All that is required is an electric supply and attention to the simple principles of using electricity safely near water.

Pool fountains

Fountains in a pool can be of many types and often come pre-fitted with submersible pumps. Select one to suit the size of pool you have and select the type of nozzle to create the sound you would like. Generally, fine jets produce minimal sound, and also tend to clog, so you need to clean the filters regularly. In a larger pool it is sensible to place the pump at the edge of the pool and run a pipe to the fountain at the centre so that servicing is easier. Remember to place the pump on a shelf clear of the debris that is likely to collect on the bottom. Nowadays you can also purchase water-bell jets and tulip jets that force water out of a disc, creating a thin film of water like an inverted sphere or bell shape. They create a different sound, a continuous rush of water rather than the splashing of a conventional fountain. Fountains that produce fine droplets and those using water bells need protected sites, patios or

LEFT: *Fountains with fine jets need protection from wind as in this Mediterranean courtyard garden.*
RIGHT: *You can enjoy the sound of a fountain without a pool, as in this Japanese garden which uses a geyser jet.*

courtyards where there is minimal wind. If you have a windy site, choose a geyser jet with a more powerful pump that forces water up a broader pipe with a foaming effect and a deeper sound. Geyser jets are unaffected by wind and are quite suitable for incorporation into formal or informal water garden designs.

You can also combine a fountain jet with an ornament, so that the water appears from a lead, terracotta, stone or fibreglass statue or bowl. Always check that what you buy is frost resistant, and that the design of the ornament is in keeping with the period of your garden and its scale. These ornaments may discolour with limescale in an alkaline area but this can be easily cleaned with a descaler, while algae can produce an attractive patina and an appearance of age.

Waterfalls

An attractive addition in an informal garden setting is the sound of small waterfalls in imitation of a natural woodland stream. This is quite easy to combine with the construction of a pool (see page 134). I would avoid using a pre-formed fibreglass moulding which is difficult to incorporate into a natural setting. It is far better to use a butyl rubber liner and to purchase one large enough for strips to be removed for lining the cascade. This is also cheaper than buying separate liners and the pieces can be welded together using a non-toxic mastic. Follow a similar procedure to that for constructing a pool and use the excavated soil to create a natural-looking graded area to take a series of pools that empty into one another. Start from the top and work up to a higher level.

Design a place for a submersible recirculating pump on a ledge just under the base of the cascade and plumb the water up to an issuing point at the top of the cascade pools using non-toxic plastic piping. Choose a pump that will provide the flow rate needed for the type of waterfall you want to hear. As a rough guide, a good fall of water over a 15cm (6in) wide lip will need a 3,000 litres (600 gallons) per hour pump. The higher the cascade or 'head' of water the more powerful the pump needs to be.

Remember that if you disturb the water with a cascade you will not be able to grow water lilies, which need a still surface.

Water features without a pool

In town gardens it is often more sensible (especially if you have small children) to have a water feature over an above-ground sealed reservoir rather than an open pool. These can be designed as cobble fountains or millstone fountains where the water bubbles up from a sealed reservoir via a submersed pump, either through the millstone or over cobbles laid on wire mesh. These features are particularly suitable for modern settings and patio gardens and do not even require an excavation. The reservoir can be formed from a lined brick or stone-built tank and you can insert the type of nozzle to create the sound you enjoy.

NB Pumps and all connections must be fully waterproofed. Ensure that the connections are earthed and that the mains connection has a circuit breaker to protect against any possibility of electric shock. Always seek expert technical advice before installing any equipment.

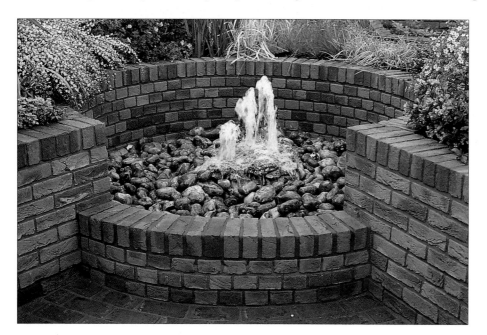

LEFT: In town gardens the sound of water can be enjoyed using a cobble fountain where brickwork is more appropriate and where there is no risk of toddlers falling in.
RIGHT: A cascade of waterfalls can be built using liners, submersible recirculating pumps of sufficient power and a good artistic sense in arranging the rockwork.

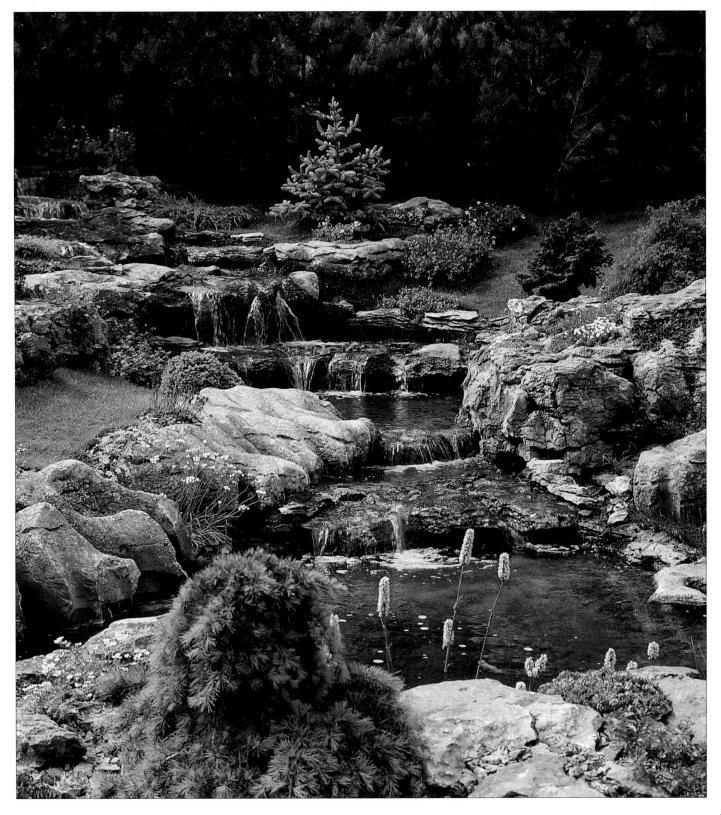

WHAT IS SCENT?

—o—

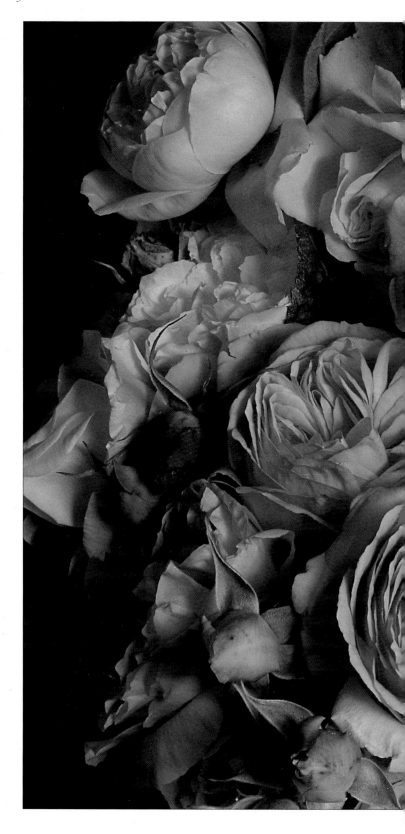

erfumed plants in the garden have a particular charm whether their fragrance is emitted from flowers or through crushing the foliage. Our appreciation of fragrance is, of course, incidental to the reason why plants produce scented essential oils. In the case of flowers this is nearly always to attract pollinators. Night-scented flowers are coloured specifically to attract night-flying insects and moths: they are mostly white, cream or very pale yellow to show up in the dark, with tubular flowers adapted to long-tongued pollinators searching for nectar, and their perfume is given off only in the cooler temperatures of the evening when the flowers open fully. Their scent is also particularly pervasive in the evening dampness and carries much further than many day scents. In nature many of these species predominate in sheltered valleys where the scent is contained, along with the pollinators, giving a clue as to how best to site them in our gardens.

Growing scented plants

Since, in general, flowers also produce perfume as a strategy to attract *instead* of producing strong flower colour, it is not an easy task to produce a brightly coloured scented garden. Rely instead on paler colours. Many modern hybrids have been bred for strong colour and have lost fragrance in the process – an example is the popular tobacco plant now available in dwarf strains of good colour, but for perfume you would need to obtain the species *Nicotiana alata* or *N. sylvestris*.

   Not all flowers produce scent that is attractive to humans. Since they are trying to attract flies or other insects they may emit the scent of decay in imitation of the decaying food sources of those insects. Many members of the arum family and tree members of the rose family (such as Hawthorn, Pyracantha and the Bird Cherry) do

Several growers, including David Austin, are breeding new roses using the old rose groups which are highly scented.

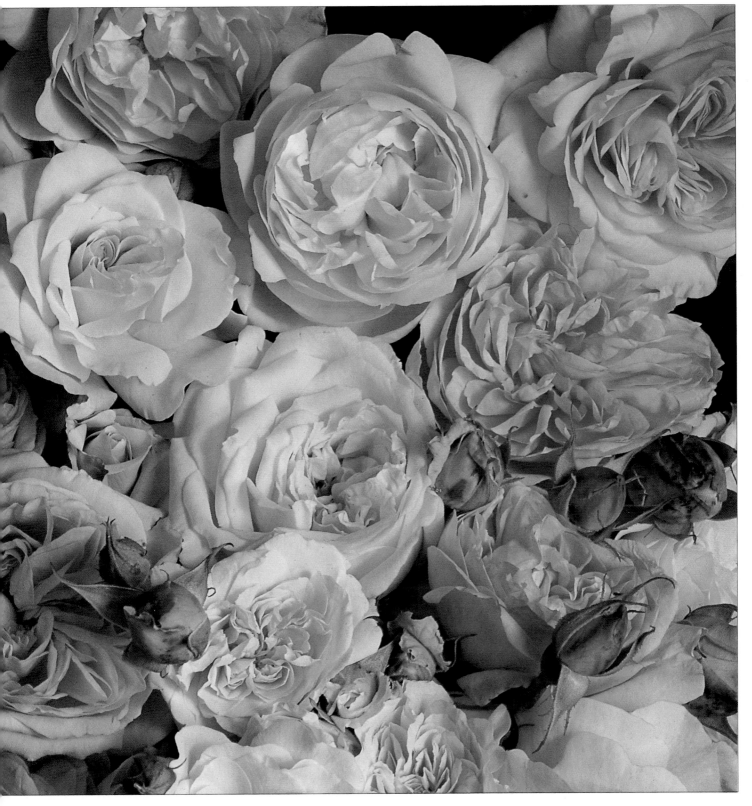

this and should always be planted well away from the house and never used as cut flowers.

Not all scent in plants is produced in flowers. Many of the essential oils are contained in the leaves and stems and are given off when the tissue is bruised or crushed. Many of these species can be used in 'touch' gardens or gardens for the blind. From the plant's point of view these substances are there to act as defence against pest attack and to repel animals from browsing. Many species originate from arid or semi-arid areas where the oils, released from their aromatic foliage by the heat of the sun, protect them from desiccation. Some tree species exude gums which are strongly antiseptic and healing of their own wounds. Many of these are used in aromatherapy and in general medicine as effective germicides – for example, Friar's Balsam, from the tropical tree *Styrax benzoin*, is used for sore throats.

Describing scent

How is the perfume of a plant described? Usually by the layperson the description is in terms of likeness to some other well-recognized scent, although there is often disagreement. The response to scent is very individual, perhaps varying with individual physiology, and perfumes vary in their effect according to dilution. In plants the response may vary according to the person's proximity to the flowers and length of inhalation. Perfumiers divide the response into several categories – top, middle and bottom notes – the top describing the initial reaction and the bottom the after-effect. These categories are sometimes also used in aromatherapy.

The healing powers of scent

That scent can have strong psychological effects has long been recognized by the perfume industry and the power of pheromones to attract is well established in animal behaviour. Analyzing the effect is more difficult. Certainly, however, response to perfume via the olfactory nerves is highly individual (said to be stronger in the dark-haired than in the fair) and smell is one of the strongest stimulators of memory. In a garden environment including plants that have particularly happy associations can be a strong antidote to depression.

Experience will show which perfumes mix well together and what density to plant so as to produce fragrance that is attractive but not overpowering – the sense of smell can be overwhelmed and become tired as easily as the palate.

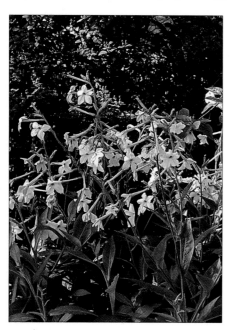

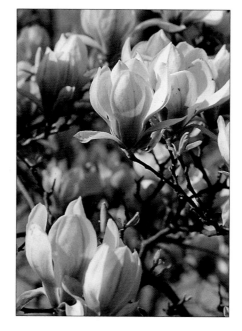

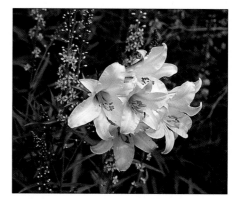

FAR LEFT: *Some fragrant plants open their flowers in the evening, as does* Nicotiana alata. LEFT: *Magnolia soulangeana is one of the lemon-scented species.* ABOVE: *Lilium regale is overpoweringly fragrant.*

A CLASSIFICATION OF PLANT SCENTS

The following table lists the generally accepted scent groups with examples of plants. It excludes the unpleasant aminoid (fishy or ammonia-like) animal-scented and indoloid (carrion-scented) groups. The most useful groups for providing attractive scent in the garden are asterisked.

Scent group	Description of scent	Fragrance due to (where known)	Examples of plants
*Aromatic	Almond Aniseed Balsam Clove Incense Pine Vanilla Violet	 Eugenol Vanilla Ionone	*Heliotropium* *Drimys winteri, Magnolia, Primula veris* *Hyacinthus orientalis* *Dianthus* *Calomeria amaranthoides* and *Liquidambar orientalis* – leaves *Pelargonium fragrans* group – leaves *Clematis montana, Laburnum* × *watereri* 'Vossii' *Lathyrus odoratus* *Crinum powellii, Iris reticulata, Reseda odorata, Violas*
Camphor	Camphor	Camphor	Leaves of *Artemisia absinthium, Laurus nobilis, Lindera benzoin, Salvia fruticosa* and *Santolina chamaecyparissus*
Eucalyptus	Eucalyptus	Eucalyptol	Leaves of *Eucalyptus, Lavandula, Myrtus, Rosmarinus* and *Thymus*
*Fruit-scented	Apple Apricot (Plum to some) Banana Orange Pineapple Plum		*Calycanthus floridus, Pelargonium odoratissimum* – leaves, *Rosa wichuraiana* *Iris graminea* *Rosa soulieana* *Pelargonium* 'Prince of Orange' – leaves, *Philadelphus, Rosa* 'Wedding Day' *Argyrocytisus battandieri, Salvia rutilans* – leaves *Freesia, Muscari neglectum*
Hay-scented		Coumarin	*Galium odoratum, Lobularia maritima*
*Heavy-scented	Aminoid-like but not unpleasant except in quantity.	Indole plus benzylacetate	*Convallaria majalis, Eucharis* × *grandiflora, Hemerocallis citrina, Lilium candidum, Lilium regale, Polianthes tuberosa, Syringa vulgaris* cultivars
*Honey-scented	Honey/musk		*Buddleja, Escallonia, Lonicera, Olearia, Sedum (Hylotelephium) spectabile*
*Lemon-scented		Citral	*Artemisia abrotanum* – leaves, *Aloysia triphylla* – leaves, *Magnolia* × *soulangiana, Oenothera odorata, Pelargonium crispum* – leaves, *Rosa bracteata*
Mint	Mint	Menthol	*Mentha* sp. – leaves
*Rose-scented	Sweet and fruity but not heavy.	Geraniol	*Paeonia suffruticosa, Pelargonium capitatum.* Many roses.

PLANNING SCENT IN YOUR GARDEN

○

If you are planning a scented garden it is wise to ensure that the perfume remains where you can gain the benefit from it. Do this by sheltering the garden from breezes that disperse scent, either by providing walls or hedges or by building a sunken garden as a separate feature within your overall design. You can also capture scent very effectively by planting scented species within a conservatory.

Placing scented plants within your garden

Plants bear their perfumes in different ways and a knowledge of this is important in deciding where to place them. For example, scents that carry can be placed at some distance from the house or from frequently used paths, or they can be massed so that their perfumes can waft from a distance. I once planted a newly designed scented garden entirely with *Nicotiana alata* for its first summer, before the structural planting was done in the autumn. The evening perfume from this carried 80 metres and brought pleasant comments from the neighbours.

Other species that waft well are all the *Mahonia* species; several lilies, especially *Lilium regale*; *Lobularia maritima* and *Aurinia saxatilis*; *Matthiola longipetala*; wallflowers *Erysimum cheiri*; the Wintersweet *Chimonanthus praecox*; *Crambe cordifolia*; *Azara microphylla*; the pineapple-scented *Argyrocytisus battandieri*; most of the *Daphne* species, especially *D. odora*; *Fritillaria imperialis* (which at the Royal Botanic Gardens, Kew, carries at least 10 metres); most of the *Lonicera* species; *Osmanthus fragrans*; all the shrubby *Philadelphus*; *Rhododendron luteum*; and most of the viburnums. Massing *Iris germanica* cultivars can provide overwhelming scent in a sunny enclosed courtyard in early summer.

On the other hand, there are plants that need a close approach before you can appreciate their fragrance and these need to be planted close to paths and frequently used routes near the house. Plants of small stature need raising to the nose, so plant them in raised beds or in stone troughs to avoid floundering on bended knee. This is particularly true of garden pinks, which also enjoy the improved drainage that goes with being raised. Other suitable plants include *Daphne cneorum eximia*, *Daphne blagayana* (this also needs leafy

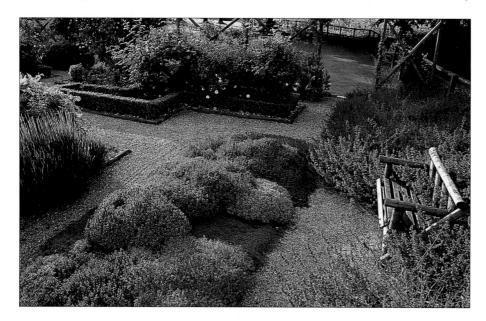

Design seats in your garden so you can enjoy the proximity of perfumes. Here, a thyme 'lawn' faces the seat. Plant roses where they can be sniffed from the path.

soil), snowdrops, *Iris danfordiae*, *Muscari* and several of the dwarf narcissi such as 'Tête-à-Tête' and *Narcissus cyclamineus*. Larger species can be grown in pots on terraces and patios or can be planted in window boxes so that their scent can be enjoyed through open windows.

Some perfumes can be so strong they can almost intoxicate, as I once learnt after planting a large tub of *Lilium regale* under the fanlight of a ground floor bedroom! You can also plant scented climbing plants on frames around a garden seat to make a bower. A medieval idea, this is particularly appropriate for scented roses, honeysuckles, jasmines and wisterias.

Some perfumes lie in the foliage of plants and need to be touched to be released. These are also best planted near a frequently used path or where you are likely to brush against them. Trees and shrubs in this category include the Mexican Orange Blossom *Choisya ternata*, *Cistus ladanifer*, *Eucalyptus*, *Aloysia triphylla*, *Myrtus* species, scented-leaved *Pelargonium* species and the lovely Incense Rose *Rosa primula* whose leaves release fragrance after rain. Small, creeping plants that can withstand being trodden on are good candidates for a crazy-paved patio or terrace where plenty of spaces have been introduced into the design. Suitable species include most thymes, the creeping camomile *Chamaemelum nobile* 'Treneague' and the wonderfully minty Corsican mint *Mentha requienii*.

Lastly, do not forget to design your scented garden for the times when it will be most used. For example, *Iris germanica* is a good choice for a garden much used in early summer. Choose evening-scented plants for a garden used at dusk and remember that in winter, scented plants such as Witch Hazel, Wintersweet and Sarcococca are best planted near the house rather than at the end of a long trek across a sodden or frozen lawn!

Scent in the conservatory

Excellent scented plants for growing in the conservatory are the climbing Star Jasmines *Trachelospermum jasminoides* and *T. asiaticum*. You could also plant the Mimosa *Acacia dealbata*, any number of the *Citrus* species, *Gardenia augusta*,

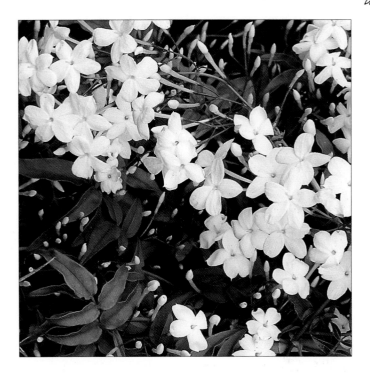

Jasminum polyanthum will have its fragrance well contained in a temperate conservatory kept frost free.

Stephanotis floribunda, *Rhododendron* x *fragrantissimum* (if you can provide lime-free soil), some of the true Jasmines such as *Jasminum polyanthum* and the richly jasmine-scented evergreen *Pittosporum tobira*. All of these will do well providing they are just kept frost-free, but if you can afford to heat to subtropical temperatures (night minimum 18°C, 60°F) then further delights become possible. Try the Amazon Lily *Eucharis* × *grandiflora* and the Tuberose *Polianthes tuberosa*, both of which can be grown in pots from bulbs or tubers. The Tuberose is a cut flower commonly used in garlands and religious offerings in Asia because of its overwhelmingly rich perfume. Try also the Jasmine used to scent Jasmine tea, *Jasminum sambac*, which has flowers like small gardenias. The scent does not carry, except in damp conditions, but you need only sniff each flower to transport yourself instantly to a tea merchant's warehouse. At the other extreme are the Hoyas, especially *Hoya carnosa*, which wafts its spicy honey scent through any warm atmosphere and is especially pungent in the evening.

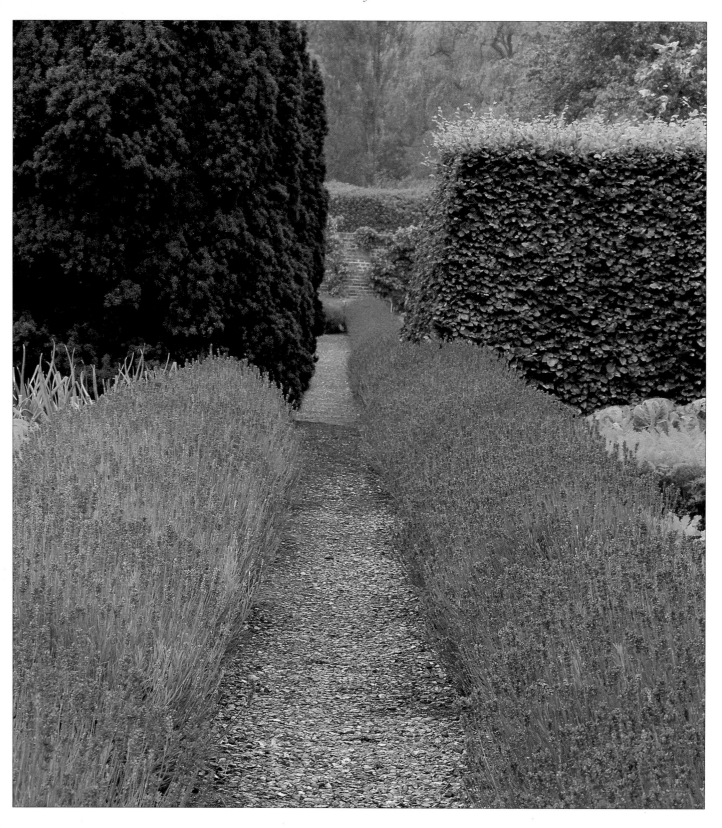

LAVENDER

Lavender is one of the best loved of the fragrant, aromatic shrubs that originate from the Mediterranean area. It has been used as a strewing herb and cultivated for its oil since the sixteenth century and produces one of the commonest oils used in aromatherapy. It also makes a worthwhile garden plant; it is quick-growing and tolerant of poor soil, providing it receives full sunlight. The dwarfer clones, such as *Lavandula* 'Hidcote' and the green-leaved *Lavandula* 'Munstead Dwarf', make excellent fragrant hedges and are a favourite for inclusion in formal herb garden designs and to line pathways.

Lavender for scent

The Romans used lavender to scent linen and also in bathing; indeed, its name may derive from the Latin verb *lavare* (to wash). Several species are grown in France and Spain, including the French lavender *Lavandula stoechas*, which is rather too tender to grow outside in Britain. Its subspecies *L. stoechas* ssp. *pedunculata* is probably the prettiest in flower. The best lavender for the production of oil is *Lavandula angustifolia*, which produces oil completely free from the taint of camphor present in other species. It is this species that is used in the English lavender industry which, along with the French, is the most famous in the world. It also has a particular link with the Chelsea Physic Garden because it was named by Philip Miller in the eighteenth century.

A range of lavender products is produced commercially using lavender oil. This is distilled by steam in a still, drawn off and then matured for a year before being blended with other oils. A huge quantity of flowers is needed to produce the essential oil – 750g (1¾lbs) weight of oil is produced from a quarter of a tonne of flowers. The oil can then be used in soaps, bath essences,

Lavender hedges create a fragrant path and enjoy the full sunlight which ripens their growth.

colognes, hand and body lotion, talc and, of course, the traditional lavender water.

You can dry lavender easily at home; the best fragrance is obtained by bunching the flowers and air drying them at low temperatures. The lavender can then be used in pomanders, made into muslin sachets to scent clothes in wardrobes and drawers and can be used on its own, or in a mixture, as pot-pourri. It also makes a fragrant confetti.

Medicinal uses of lavender

Lavender has been used medicinally since the time of the English herbalist John Gerard (1545-1612) who recommended it for 'panting and passion of the heart' and giddiness. Its oil was a constituent of 'palsy drops', officially recognized in the British *Pharmacopoeia* as a treatment for palpitations. In herbal medicine lavender is used to treat infection and to relieve aches and pains. It is used as a relaxant in aromatherapy and is reputedly excellent in reducing stress-induced headache, indigestion and irritability, and is helpful in ensuring peaceful sleep.

How to grow lavender

Plant young plants between early autumn and early spring in well-drained soil in full sun. Set plants 22–30cm (9–12in) apart for hedges. Trim old flowerheads from the plants in late summer if not picked earlier for drying. Cut all plants back in early spring to encourage bushy growth. Plan to replace plants after about five to eight years as lavenders are not long-lived. Propagate by taking 7.5cm (3in) cuttings of non-flowering shoots in late summer and rooting them in a coir/sand mixture in a cold frame.

Lavender can also be propagated from seed but the species hybridize and clones do not come true by this method. *L.* 'Hidcote', one of the best lavenders, and *L.* 'Munstead', both forms of *L. angustifolia*, are best vegetatively propagated by cuttings, and this is quite easy to do.

ESSENTIAL OILS AND AROMATHERAPY

Aromatherapy is curative treatment based on the use of essential oils derived from plants. Its history is pre-Christian and the principal ancient cultures that practised it were the Chinese, Egyptians, Greeks and Romans, all of whom used aromatic oils, although the oils were probably infused rather than distilled.

Aromatic oils of the ancients

The 'royal gifts' of frankincense and myrrh given to the child Christ attest the importance of plant aromas in religious practices. *Boswellia carteri* and *Commiphora myrrha* are both resinous trees of the semi-desert areas of North East Africa and have a long tradition of use. Incense was used in Egypt on state occasions and the pyramids have yielded the remains of ointments and oils. From Egypt, the use of aromatic plants passed to the Greeks, and thence to the Arabs who first invented the process of distilling essential oils from the resinous woody species of their homelands. Some sources have credited the discovery to the Persian physician Avicenna (AD 980–1037). The perfumes of Arabia were as sought after by the Crusaders as were the 'spices of the Orient' in the seventeenth-century exploration of the Far East. For the southern Europeans the equivalent of the resinous trees of Arabia were their native aromatics such as rosemary, lavender and thyme, and oils from these plants were sold to the general population by druggists and apothecaries.

The popularity of aromatherapy today derives from work done almost entirely by the Frenchmen Gattefosse and Valnet and, some of the greatest aromatherapy houses are French.

Using essential oils

Aromatherapy is mostly empirically based – that is, the effects of oils are determined by observation. However, some aromatherapists subscribe to complex theories concerning the way the oils are absorbed and then heal via meridians in the body. It is not necessary to believe in these theories to enjoy aromatic oils from plants, though anyone using them regularly should consult a trained aromatherapist, as some oils can be toxic.

Essential oils are absorbed through the skin and by inhalation. The most popular use is through massage (where the oil or blend of oils is mixed with a carrier oil), in bathing and also by creams, lotions and compresses. Many of these oils are expensive because a large quantity of plant material is necessary to produce a small drop of oil. Some are also the products of tropical species, particularly the exotic and supposedly aphrodisiac, and so cannot be grown outdoors in a temperate climate. Many others, however, are derived from plants that can be grown in an 'aromatherapy garden' for your own interest and delight, though you are unlikely to be able to grow enough for commercial cropping.

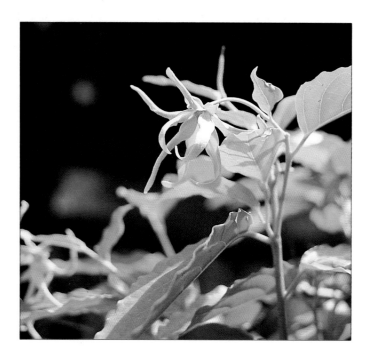

Ylang-Ylang is an aphrodisiac oil which is produced from the flowers of Cananga odorata.

A TABLE OF AROMATHERAPY OILS

The following table lists the oils and the botanical name of the species from which they are obtained. All, except the tropical species, can be grown outside but it is best to take those that are marked with an asterisk (first column) into a cool greenhouse over winter. In general, aromatherapy oils are safe providing they are applied to the skin in a carrier oil and not neat. However, do heed the warnings given.

Common Name	Botanical Name	Warning	Reputed Effect
TEMPERATE OILS			
Basil*	*Ocimum basilicum*	●■	Uplifting, stimulating.
Bergamot	*Citrus bergamia*	✳	Refreshing, analgesic, anti-depressant, antiseptic.
Camomile	*Chamaemelum nobile*		Refreshing, analgesic, anti-depressant, febrifuge.
Cedarwood	*Cedrus atlantica*		Sedative.
Clary-sage	*Salvia sclarea*	●	Warming, aphrodisiac, anti-depressant, calming.
Cypress	*Cupressus sempervirens*		Refreshing, deodorant.
Eucalyptus	*Eucalyptus globulus*		Warming, antiseptic, expectorant, febrifuge.
Geranium*	*Pelargonium odoratissimum*		Refreshing, relaxing, anti-depressant.
Juniper	*Juniperus communis*	●	Refreshing, stimulating, detoxifying.
Lavender	*Lavandula angustifolia*		Refreshing, relaxing, analgesic, antiseptic.
Lemon*	*Citrus limonum*	■ ✳	Refreshing, stimulating.
Lemon verbena*	*Aloysia triphylla*	■ ✳	Antiseptic, insect-repellent.
Marjoram	*Origanum majorana*	●	Warming, analgesic, relaxing.
Melissa	*Melissa officinalis*	■	Uplifting, anti-depressant, febrifuge.
Neroli*	*Citrus aurantium*	✳	Very relaxing, anti-depressant, aphrodisiac.
Peppermint	*Mentha piperata*	●■	Cooling, stimulating.
Petigrain*	*Citrus bigaradia*		Refreshing, anti-depressant.
Pine Needle	*Pinus sylvestris*		Refreshing, antiseptic.
Rose	*Rosa centifolia/damascena*	●	Relaxing, soothing, anti-depressant, aphrodisiac.
Rosemary	*Rosmarinus officinalis*	●▲	Invigorating, analgesic, antiseptic.
Tarragon*	*Artemisia dracunculus*		Warming.
Thyme	*Thymus vulgaris*	■▲	Antiseptic.
TROPICAL OILS			
Benzoin	*Styrax benzoin*		Warming, relaxing, expectorant, wound-healing.
Black pepper	*Piper nigrum*		Stimulating, warming.
Frankincense	*Boswellia carteri*		Relaxing, reviving, astringent.
Ginger	*Zingiber officinale*		Warming, digestive.
Jasmine	*Jasminum grandiflorum*		Soothing, anti-depressant, aphrodisiac.
Lemongrass	*Cymbopogon citratus*	■	Tonic, refreshing.
Myrrh	*Commiphora myrrha*	●	Cooling, tonic, anti-inflammatory, fungicidal.
Patchouli	*Pogostemon patchouli*		Relaxing.
Sandalwood	*Santalum album*		Relaxing, anti-depressant, antiseptic, aphrodisiac.
Tea Tree	*Melaleuca alternifolia*	■	Antiseptic, antiviral, febrifuge, tonic.
Ylang-Ylang	*Cananga odorata*		Relaxing, aphrodisiac, anti-depressant.

KEY

● Do not use in pregnancy   ✳ Do not use where skin is exposed to strong sunlight
■ Do not use on sensitive skins   ▲ Do not use with high blood pressure

THE STREWING OF HERBS AND SCENTING OF THE AIR

Dried fragrant plants were used throughout Europe in medieval times and during the sixteenth and seventeenth centuries as the equivalent to today's air fresheners. Damp air rose from earthen floors, so herbs that gave fragrance when stepped upon were in much demand. Commonly used species were camomile, lavender, hyssop, sage, thyme, costmary, meadowsweet, basil, balm and the scented rush *Acorus calamus*. John Gerard, the English herbalist, mentioned the practice of strewing herbs on the floor, and all English monarchs up to George IV had a 'Strewer of Herbs' as an official appointment.

Protection against disease

There was some appreciation that certain aromatic herbs protected against disease. Rue, rosemary and thyme were often carried in the street to protect against plague or worn by judges as a defence against being infected by those brought before them. Modern aromatherapists have investigated the germicidal properties of essential oils and claim that the most effective are those of cinnamon, lavender, clove, thyme, rosemary and geranium, along with attar of rose petals. Part of their effectiveness may also have been due to their repelling insects, the vectors of disease.

Roses were also used extensively in perfumery, particularly the petals of *Rosa × damascena*, most likely introduced from the Middle East by the Crusaders, and those of *Rosa gallica* 'Officinalis', widely known as the Apothecaries' Rose because it retained its fragrance longest and was used in medicine as well as in perfumery. Otherwise known as the Provins rose, because it was grown around the town of Provins in France, French apothecaries used the flowers to produce rose water, rose vinegar and rose-honey conserves, all of which were used therapeutically.

Scenting and fumigation

Sixteenth-century houses contained herb and still rooms where women laboured to produce medicinal products for the household. The aim was to produce 'sweet waters' from distilled essential oils, such as rose water, violet water and lavender water so that they could be used to scent clothes or sprinkle around rooms. Pomanders made out of porcelain, silver or dried fruits were carried attached to belts or as necklaces, and clothes were often stored in chests made of fragrant woods such as cedar or sandalwood.

Before the germ theory of disease it was widely believed that 'foul and pestilential airs' caused disease. Thus itinerant perfumiers were called in to fumigate houses with fragrant woods (usually juniper or Scots pine) before evaporating rose water into the atmosphere. Other species used were *Inula conyzae*, elecampane, angelica and the roots of *Rhodiola rosea*. Snuffs of finely ground tobacco were also used to protect from plague. Lavender, cinnamon, clove and bergamot oils were all used to impart protection into the snuff.

Pot-pourri

Today the art of strewing has died out, but essential oils are still used to fumigate with more modern methods that include evaporation from rings heated on electric light bulbs. The equivalent of many of the practices which reached their height as a reaction to the poor hygiene of medieval Europe is the humble pot-pourri.

Many pot-pourris can be bought cheaply which use wood shavings as a base into which fragrant oils are impregnated. To make a true pot-pourri with leaf, flower and spice ingredients takes time and considerable adjustment of moisture level using the traditional orris root and salt.

A RECIPE FOR A ROSE POT-POURRI

Petals of 40 strongly scented roses (for example Rosa
centifolia *varieties)*
Handful of lavender flowers
Handful of lemon verbena leaves
Handful of mint leaves
Handful of calendula and delphinium
flowers (for colour)
12g (½oz) oil of lavender
12g (½oz) oil of geranium
A few cinnamon sticks
25g (1oz) ground nutmeg
25g (1oz) cloves (whole)
25g (1oz) coriander seeds
100g (4oz) salt
100g (4oz) orris root powder

Collect the rose petals when no moisture is on them and allow them to dry quickly in an airy place away from bright light. When dry, layer them with salt in an airtight jar. Shake daily.

Dry the other leaves and flowers and add to the roses after five days of drying.

Add the oils to the orris powder and then add the spices. Add the dry flowers and leave for four weeks in a covered bowl, stirring now and then. Adjust the moisture level with more salt (to dry) or more orris (to moisten). Decant into bowls for use. The pot-pourri can be freshened with rose oil as needed.

Pot-pourri is a modern equivalent of the medieval 'strewing herbs', both used to perfume rooms.

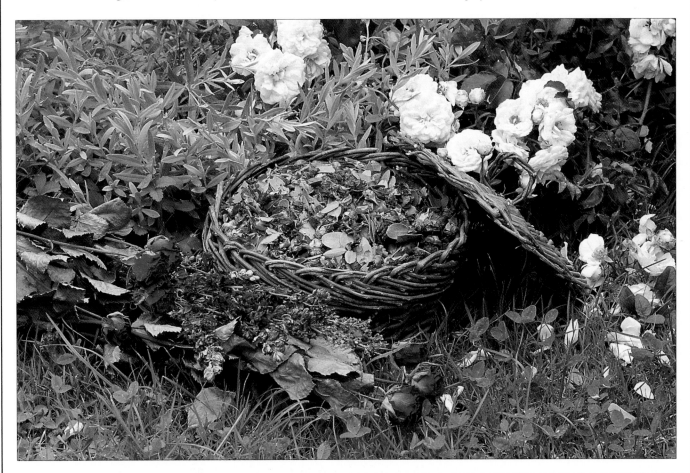

THE TEXTURE OF PLANTS

Certain plants are simply delightful to touch and enjoy, even if just at a particular time of year, such as spring when beech unfurls its delicately soft leaves before they toughen up as summer progresses.

Leaves

Leaves display an enormous variety of textures. Some plants, such as *Crambe* and *Macleaya*, have waxy leaves; others have huge smooth leaves, like *Canna*, or rubbery leaves like water lilies. Each have their own quality.

In early summer some plants, such as the moisture-loving *Rodgersia* species, have a finely quilted feel as the leaves expand. Then there are plants which are simply furry. Examples of these are some of the verbascums, the beautiful (but frost-tender) *Buddleja crispa*, and *Lavandula lanata* (*lanata* meaning woolly). My two personal favourites are *Salvia argentea* and *Pelargonium tomentosum*. The salvia is a delight in mid and late spring when its rounded leaves are deeply white-felted, an effect that changes totally as the flower spike emerges in early summer and the leaves become coarser and greener. This species is a biennial and seeds itself quite freely. *Pelargonium tomentosum* is peppermint scented, an added joy as you touch the leaves that are as soft as mohair.

There are plants (mainly in the succulent family Aizoaceae) which are cold to the touch. They include several of the mesembryanthemums, and the Hottentot Fig *Carpobrotus edulis*. These plants are popularly and appropriately called 'Ice plants', and are especially pleasant to touch on a hot day.

Some plants are sticky to touch or produce waxes to protect themselves from the heat of the sun in Mediterranean climates. *Cistus* are an example of a genus which produces a fragrant wax called 'labdanum' after a cool night which can be collected and used medicinally in bronchitis. The buds of most cistus species are attractive to touch and smell.

Barks

The barks of some trees feel quite unusual. Try touching the bark of the Cork Oak *Quercus suber* with your eyes closed. This is the Mediterranean tree from whose bark corks for bottles are made, and it is deeply fissured. Some of the snakebark maples such as *Acer davidii* ssp. *grosseri*, *Acer capillipes* or *Acer davidii* are interesting to touch. Then there is the contrasting feel of trees that shed their bark, such as *Acer griseum*, *Luma apiculata* or *Betula papyrifera* the Paper Birch, or even those that mainly stay intact such as *Prunus serrula*, whose stem gleams like polished mahogany and is as pleasing and slippery to the touch as a finely turned boardroom table.

Flowers and seedheads

In summer it is often a real pleasure to walk around a garden and touch petals as they expand, particularly those with a satiny sheen. Try touching the petals of *Crinum* lilies or any of the American daisies

Scented Pelargonium tomentosum *is soft to touch.*

such as *Coreopsis* or *Cosmos*. Even dahlia petals are a delight. Run your hand up the inflorescence of a grass to feel its silkiness or cup your hand around the perfect sphere of an *Allium* or *Echinops* flower. Lay your palm onto the flatness of an *Achillea filipendulina* seedhead; no wonder the cultivar name is 'Gold Plate'!

Seedheads can have an extraordinary quality of lightness as you touch them and the seeds disperse. They can be scaly like *Centaurea* or curiously papery like many of the 'everlasting' flowers that can be kept through the winter.

Certain plants almost invite you to investigate them by touch, from the universal appeal of *Antirrhinum* flowers, which gape on being squeezed, to the delight of species that disperse their seed explosively. From the *Impatiens* that burst their pods, to Honesty *Lunaria rediviva* that holds its black seeds between silky membranes, these are plants to explore and enjoy by the sense of touch.

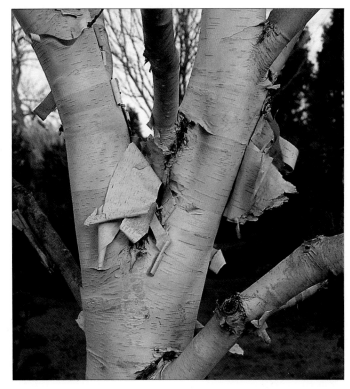

RIGHT: Betula papyrifera, *a birch which sheds its tactile bark.*

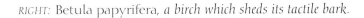

PLANTS TO ENJOY TOUCHING

Botanical name/Common name	Maximum height and spread	Comment
Acer capillipes Snakebark Maple	7.5 × 6m (25 × 20ft)	Striated bark.
Acer griseum Paperbark Maple	5 × 3m (16 × 10ft)	Flaking and peeling bark. Slow-growing.
Achillea filipendulina 'Gold Plate'	2 × 1m (6 × 3ft)	Very flat flowers. Good for drying.
Allium giganteum	1–1.5 × 0.3m (3–5 × 1ft)	Dense globular flowerheads.
Antirrhinum majus 'Nanum Compactum'	30–60 × 25cm (1–2ft × 10in)	Best grown as half-hardy annuals.
Betula papyrifera Paper Birch	9 × 4.5m (30 × 15ft)	Peeling white bark.
Buddleja crispa	3 × 2.5m (10 × 8ft)	White-felted leaves and stems.
Canna × generalis Canna Lily	1.5 × 0.45m (5 × 1½ft)	Produces satiny leaves. Not winter-hardy.
Centaurea dealbata Cornflower	60 × 60cm (2 × 2ft)	Attractive seedheads.
Coreopsis tinctoria	60–90 × 20cm (2–3ft × 8in)	Profuse flowers with satiny petals.
Cosmos bippinatus cultivars	1.2 × 0.45m (4 × 1½ft)	Profuse flowers with satiny petals. Best in poor soil.
Crambe maritima	60 × 90cm (2 × 3ft)	Very waxy, grey leaves.
Crinum × powellii	1.2 × 1m (4 × 3ft)	Waxy petals. Best in warm gardens.
Echinops ritro Globe Thistle	1.2 × 0.6m (4 × 2ft)	Perfectly globular seedheads.
Lavandula lanata	60 × 90cm (2 × 3ft)	Woolly shoots and leaves. Only for warm gardens.
Macleaya cordata Plume Poppy	1.5–2 × 1m (5–7 × 3ft)	Waxy leaves, softly plume-like flowerheads.
Quercus suber Cork Oak	6 × 3.5m (20 × 12ft)	Rugged bark, the source of cork.
Rodgersia podophylla	1.2 × 0.75m (4 × 2½ft)	Quilted young leaves. Needs moist soil.
Salvia argentea Silver Sage	60 × 60cm (2 × 2ft)	Densely white-haired leaves. Self-seeds.

A GARDEN FOR THE PARTIALLY SIGHTED

○

People who are partially sighted, like most people with disabilities, want access to areas of life that others take for granted. This is no less true of gardening and garden visiting.

Basic improvements

There are many practical ways in which the visually impaired can be helped to garden for themselves and in which their access to gardens can be improved. This opens gardening as a therapeutic activity as well as one for enjoyment. For example, the partially sighted can often see tools and pots that are painted yellow. (This is why international warning signs are painted in yellow, because they can be seen in reduced light and visibility.) Buying pots in different shapes and using this as a system to differentiate young plants is helpful. Braille printers will print out the names of plants on to plastic self-adhesive tape which can be applied to standard plant labels, or on to metal for more permanent labelling. Spacing tools can be made fairly easily to assist in planting out young plants.

If you are designing a private garden for a partially sighted person or wanting to improve access to a garden often visited by the blind, there are several points to consider. People who use tapping sticks need sizeable kerbs to feel their way around and these should be substantial enough not to act as trips for others. Alternatively, a rope fixed at hand height makes a useful guide to follow around a garden. Steps can be replaced with shallow ramps and you can indicate changes in level by using a change of paving texture that is significant enough to be felt through shoes.

Planting for touch, taste, sound and scent

There are many plants you can use to encourage enjoyment by the use of the senses of touch, taste, hearing and smell. With touch, it is obviously important to avoid plants that are thorny or that are likely to produce an allergic reaction (for example, rue). The blind need to feel free to touch safely and explore. Plant in groups that are large enough to withstand a little damage. Use plants with furry leaves, such as *Stachys byzantina*, and especially the wide range of aromatic herbs and scented-leaved pelargoniums that release their scent only when touched. As most of these are low-growing plants, build raised beds so that they can be handled easily. You can put a guide rail around such a bed with braille labels incorporated to encourage touching and describe what can be experienced at what month. Plants that can be safely tasted, such as the culinary herbs, can be planted in raised beds and labelled similarly.

There are many 'Gardens for the Blind' that have been planted with scented species for their special enjoyment. It is important to make sure that such a garden is sheltered, warm and therefore likely to contain the perfumes. Plant in masses to increase the chance of scent carrying, especially near seats. Remember also to choose species for the months when the garden is most heavily used and also for the time of day. There is little use planting night-scented species if the garden is hardly used after dusk, but every reason to plant them under windows likely to be opened on a warm night.

Encourage birds into the garden so that their song can be enjoyed. Do this by providing bird tables and nestboxes and also by providing the type of plants that form their natural food sources (see table on page 145). Lastly, consider adding a safe water feature, such as the type of sealed-reservoir fountains described on page 100. This can add the enjoyment of the sound of water without the risk an open pool would obviously pose for a partially sighted person.

This garden uses a safe, sealed-reservoir fountain and a guide rail where plants can be named in braille.

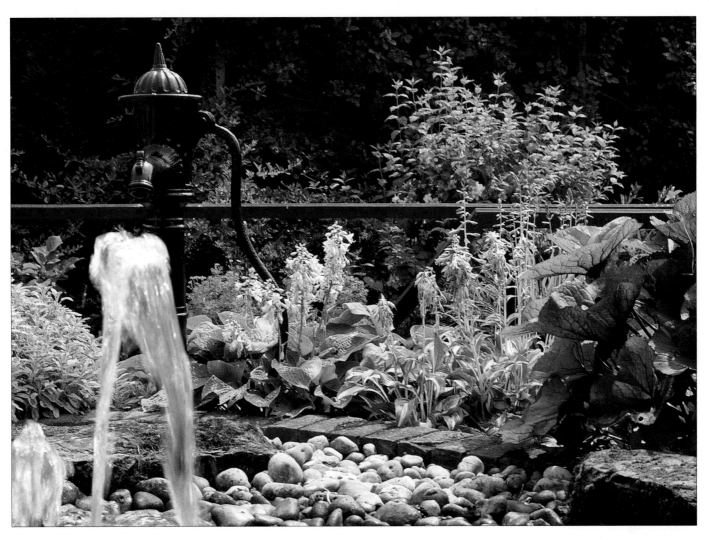

HIGHLY SCENTED PLANTS

Botanical name	Maximum height and spread	Comment
Daphne odora 'Aureo Marginata'	1.8 × 1.8m (6 × 6ft)	Scent carries well.
Dianthus 'Mrs Sinkins'	30 × 45cm (1 × 1½ft)	Replace with younger plants every few years.
Heliotropium cultivars	30 × 30cm (1 × 1ft)	Smells of cooked cherry pie.
Hyacinthus orientalis cultivars	23 × 20cm (9 × 8in)	Plant massed.
Lilium regale	1.2m × 23cm (4ft × 9in)	Best lily for perfume.
Lonicera japonica 'Halliana'	6–9 × 6m (18–30 × 18ft)	The sweetest smelling honeysuckle.
Nicotiana alata	1 × 0.30m (3 × 1ft)	Plant massed. Evening scented.
Philadelphus cultivars	from 60 × 60cm to 3 × 2.5m (2 × 2ft to 10 × 8ft)	Lovely but short flowering season.
Rosa 'Comte de Chambord'	1.2 × 1m (4 × 3ft)	Very heady scent.
Rosmarinus officinalis	1.2 × 1m (4 × 3ft)	For touching.
Syringa vulgaris cultivars	3.5 × 3m (12 × 10ft)	Lovely but short flowering season.

PLANT TREATMENTS TO MAKE
YOU FEEL GOOD

T here are many beauty treatments that use plant oils or plant fragrances to induce a sense of natural well-being. Some of these are used in general aromatherapy (see page 110) and others are used in massage, facials and beauty treatments of all kinds.

Massage

There is some evidence that plant essential oils assist in cell regeneration and healing when applied to the skin. However, they must be diluted in a vegetable oil to avoid skin irritation; almond, sunflower, grapeseed or peach kernel oil can be used as carriers and only a 3 per cent concentration of the essential oil is needed. Firm massage strokes warm the skin and assist the penetration of the oil, a process which takes at least ten minutes and can be well over an hour. Blood circulation improves and increased stimulation of the lymphatic system helps to remove toxins (and particularly lactic acid) that have built up in the muscles causing the familiar stiffness and pain. Lactic acid is also built up after strong exercise; that is why athletes need massage as well as tense office workers!

Massage also reconnects you by touch to other people, which in itself releases tension, helps human bonding, improves self-esteem and all that we recognize as good in the phrases 'the healing touch' and 'the laying on of hands'.

Several plant oils, such as almond, apricot kernel and wheatgerm, have vitamins which can be absorbed by the skin. Sweet almond oil contains vitamins F and E which assist nail growth and so is good for the hands. Apricot kernel oil contains vitamin A which softens hardened skin on the feet and wheatgerm oil contains vitamin B. Lotions that contain cooling peppermint oil are also good for tired, aching feet.

Other plant products are used in the massage process, particularly in self-massage. One of these is the loofah, which is the dried fibrous residue of the cucumber relative *Luffa cylindrica*. Loofahs can be used in the bath or shower to remove dead skin and also to improve the blood circulation and drainage of the lymphatic system. Brush up the arms, down the neck and shoulders to the back and stomach, and then start again at the

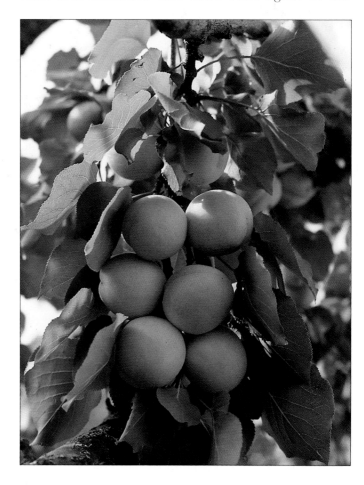

ABOVE: *The kernels of apricots produce an oil rich in vitamin A, one of the best for massage.*

toes, up the legs and over the thighs. In this way you are working towards the heart, an essential feature of good massage technique. You can also use brushes made from Sisal *Agave sisalana.* Always wash out loofahs and sisal products in warm and then cold water to prevent them degenerating too rapidly and becoming discoloured.

Using plant oils and fragrances to pamper yourself at the end of a day can be a really pleasant way of improving skin tone, enhancing your self-esteem and reconnecting you to the natural world.

A PEPPERMINT FOOT MASSAGE

Buy some unscented massage lotion. Pour some into a bowl and add two drops of oil of peppermint. Mix well and apply to one foot at a time. Commence massaging the toes. Pull them gently and rotate them one by one, then move up the foot towards the ankle using the whole hand to massage. Massage under the ball of the foot, up into the instep and finally the heel and up into the ankle. End by using both hands over the whole foot from toe to ankle in smooth, continuous strokes. Notice how the blood is circulating, yet the skin feels cooler. Repeat the method with the other foot.

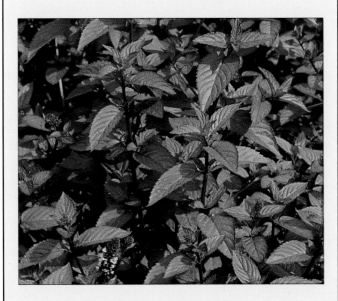

Mentha piperata is the source of peppermint oil.

A BEDTIME FACIAL

Remove any make-up and warm your skin by giving it a facial sauna over a bowl of boiling water for five minutes. Use a towel over your head to keep the steam around your face. Dry your face and then massage in wheatgerm oil into which you have mixed two drops of 3 per cent diluted oil of lavender and of rose. Use the fingers of both hands and massage outwards from the bridge of the nose, above and under the eyes, outwards across the forehead and cheeks and outwards from the chin along the jaw line. Finally, massage the neck with downward movements of the palm of the hands towards the shoulders and back.

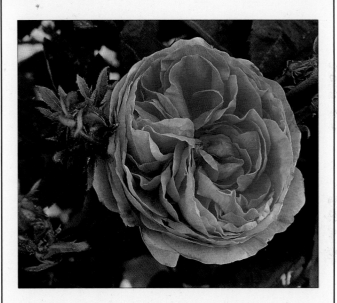

Rosa centifolia petals are cropped to produce rose oil.

A SOOTHING STEAM FACIAL

Fill a bowl with boiling water and add five drops of peppermint oil. Cover your head with a towel and lean over the water inhaling the vapour and allowing it to spread over your skin. It will cool tired muscles.

NB Do not use if you are using homoeopathic remedies as peppermint oil is said to antidote them.

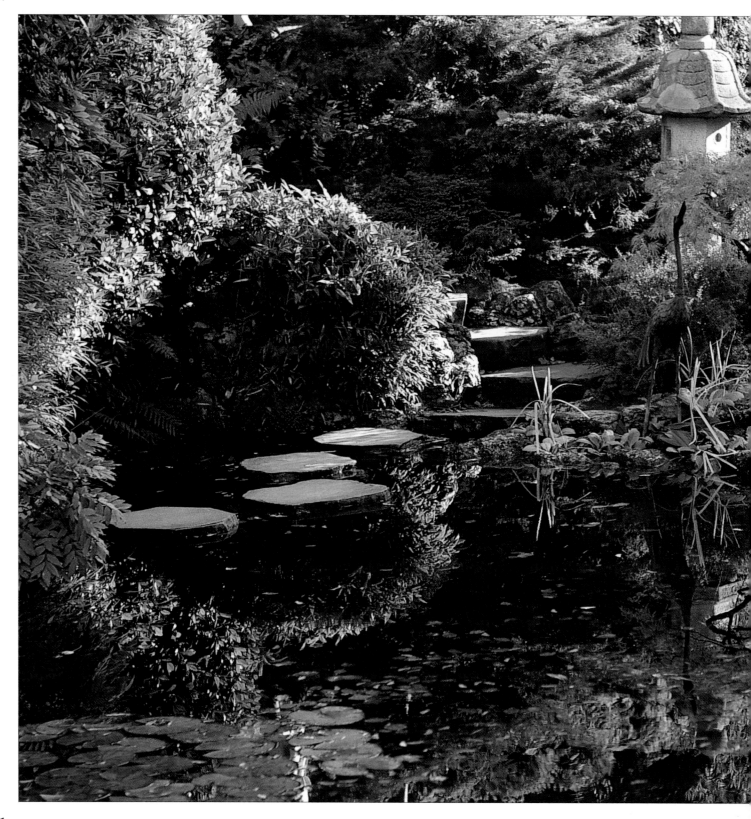

CHAPTER FOUR

A SPIRITUAL HAVEN

○

The search for paradise

Throughout history the garden has held a central place in the spiritual quest for paradise and appears in most of the world's great religions. Our own gardens are sanctuaries in a similar way, bringing refreshment, a place of growth, change and peace. Unlike nature, these gardens are ours to design to express our personal needs for a haven. Looking at the great traditions of garden design can give you ideas for your own garden and the particular effect you wish to contrive, whether formal and contained, romantic and wild, eccentric or bizarre. The garden can be a place of self-expression which can be unique to each individual, yours to labour or to relax in, a private place according to your own needs. If your life is dominated by timetables and demands imposed by others, the garden is the chance to have your own space, a personal piece of paradise. Some key species of plants that will help you design your own special haven are illustrated on pages 122–23.

The Japanese reverence for nature is expressed in their gardens – places of tranquillity, reflection and often sites for symbolic spiritual journeys.

PLANTS WHICH CONNECT YOU WITH A SPIRITUAL HAVEN

Certain flowers in religious art are symbols of purity and peace, while others attract wildlife as if into the Garden of Eden. Shrubs and trees used in some of our great traditions of garden design can remind us of how gardens are mirrors of the social and psychological needs of their age as well as of ours today. Here is a selection for your garden.

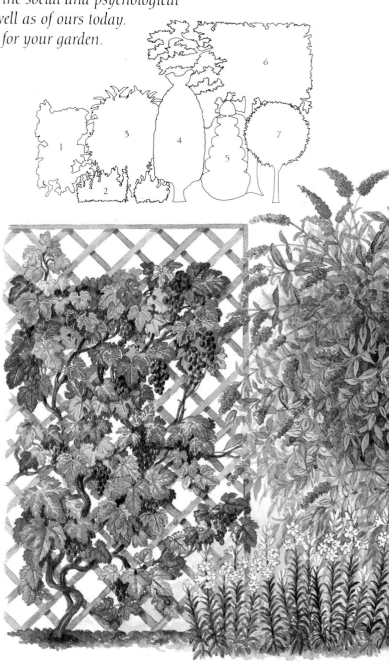

1. The Grape Vine *Vitis vinifera*, source of fruit. Plant in autumn; spur prune to obtain a good yield.
2. The Madonna Lily *Lilium candidum*, symbol of purity in Christian religious art. Plant the bulbs between autumn and spring.
3. The Butterfly bush *Buddleja davidii* and its cultivars flower profusely and attract a wide range of butterflies in late summer. Prune hard in early spring to obtain flower on the tips of the summer's subsequent growth.
4. The Common Box *Buxus sempervirens* makes an excellent, pollution-resistant, species for pruning into topiary. Trim in late summer.
5. English Yew *Taxus baccata* can be trimmed to sharp-edged lines. Do this in late summer.
6. The Hupeh Rowan *Sorbus hupehensis* produces white fruits which greatly attract bird life as well as provide welcome autumn colour.
7. The Sweet Bay *Laurus nobilis* can be trimmed to a mop-headed formal shape. Do this with secateurs in mid summer.

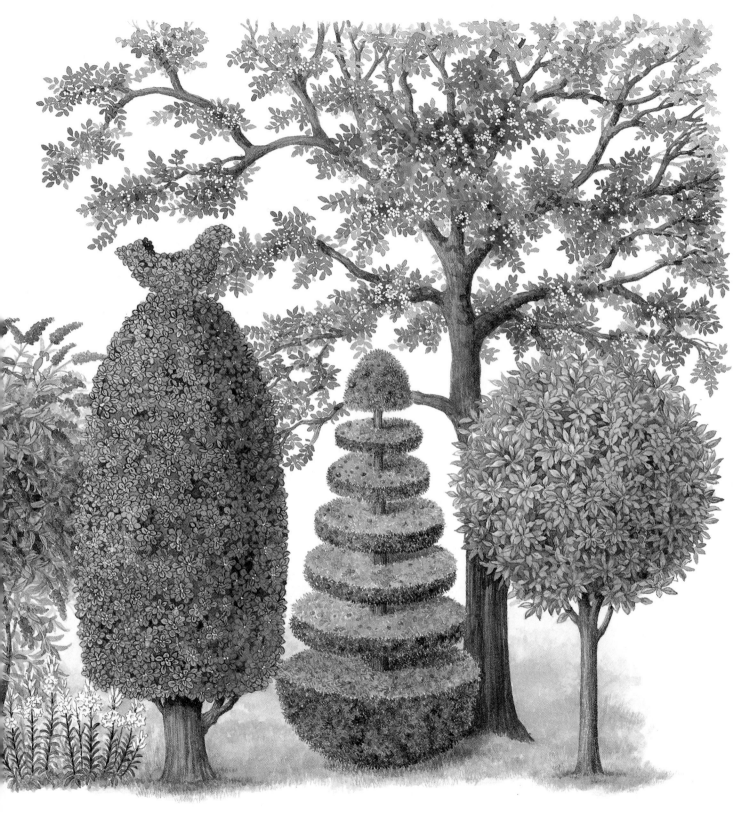

THE SECRET GARDEN

— o —

The concept of a hidden, enclosed garden kept apart for secret solitude and refreshment has been repeated through many cultures since pre-Biblical times and seems to command a strong emotional appeal.

Many people know the phrase *The Secret Garden* from the children's book of that name by Frances Hodgson Burnett. The story tells of a garden of delight turned into a garden of sorrow by the death of a beloved wife thrown from a swing when a bough breaks. The garden is locked up and neglected until found by chance. It becomes a source of joy and healing to the disabled and sickly daughter of the owner, and in her urge to restore the garden again to its former beauty, her father overcomes his grief, she recovers her health and the garden flowers once again.

This powerful image of a garden loved, then lost, and found again, is a retelling of the Biblical story of the loss of Eden and the urge to find Paradise again. But it is not only a Christian image. 'Paradise' is derived from the Persian word 'pairidaeza' meaning 'enclosure' and in the Islamic world the Koran promises the faithful that the 'Gardens of Paradise shall be their hospitality, therein to dwell forever, desiring no removal from them'. Traditionally, Islamic gardens were calm, cool sanctuaries from the hot and dusty countryside, a place of healing and, like oases, always full of water, the source of life. They portrayed a vision of what heaven would be like, and one's presence in the garden a foretaste of delights to come in paradise.

The idea of an enclosed squared garden with a pool at its centre is one that also appears in Buddhist mandalas. These were intended as meditational tools, easing the centring of the self and focusing energy on the still centre at the axis of the whirling universe, the point from which all creativity emerges.

In the medieval period the Christian religion put a particular interpretation on the whole concept of an enclosed garden. The *Hortus conclusus* was a secret garden associated with the Virgin Mary. The garden represented her virginity, and its flowers and fruits the flowering of her virginity. It was paradise found, as against the paradise lost of the lost Eden and therefore represented redemption. These gardens were often rose gardens, frequently with water features and pleasant arbours, and always enclosed, usually by a wall, sometimes by a hedge. Occasionally they were courtyard gardens, particularly in monasteries and convents where traditionally designs were inward looking.

In the fifteenth century, the Italian Renaissance added its own interpretation to the secret garden or *giardino segreto*. Such gardens remained separate, as areas intended for relaxation and privacy but less strongly enclosed. Most of the villa gardens were built in the hills above the heat (and plagues) of nearby cities such as Florence and part of their charm were the views and the breezes they commanded. The Villa Medici has its *giardino segreto* overlooking Florence, while that at the Villa Gamberaia looks over the Florentine hillsides with a belvedere or raised terrace at one end. The villas of Frascati developed quite grandly ornamented secret gardens, though always keeping the element of a predominantly enclosed 'garden within a garden'.

Today, the idea of a garden as a secret sanctuary still commands a lot of appeal. Perhaps this refers to a strong need for privacy in an overcrowded society. Most gardeners feel that the garden becomes 'theirs' in the evening when they are alone in it, as if the basic patterns of growth speak to them silently, particularly when the garden is recovering from the heat of the day. These are surely images of regeneration, of recovery and of healing.

Secret gardens are enclosed, private places, symbolic of the self. There is usually a gate or door and one certain imperative – you must find the key.

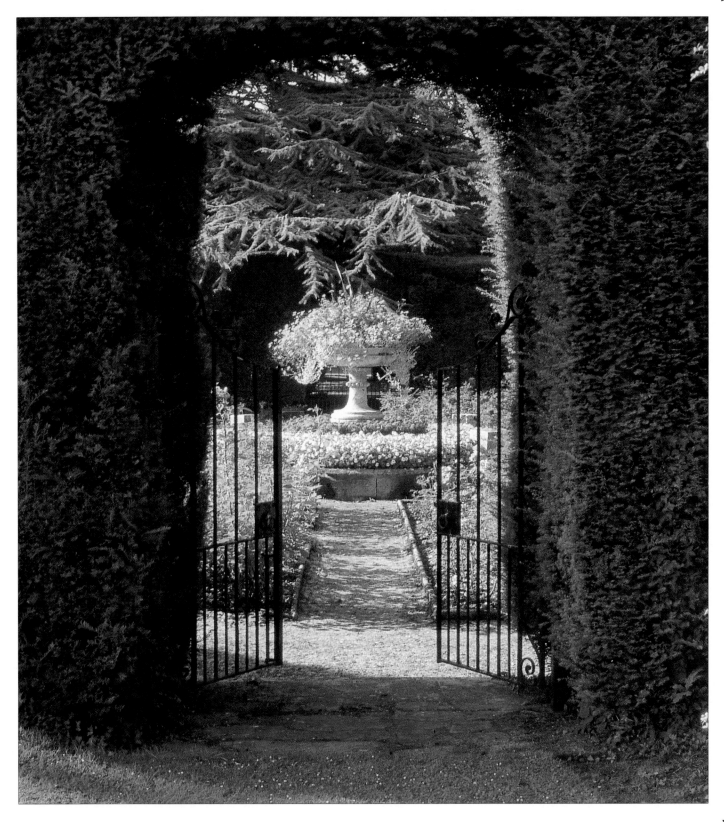

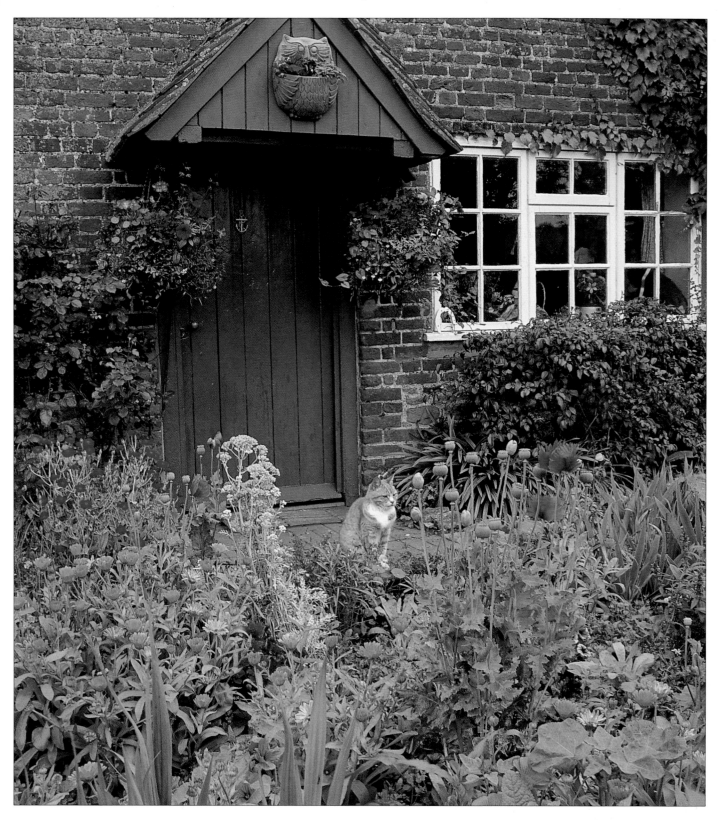

GARDEN DESIGN: NATURE AND ORDER

In modern-day domestic gardens design can play an important role in our own view of the natural world and how we wish to interact with it. It can affirm our personality in a healing sense, giving us a chance to create a living space just as we wish it to be.

The formal garden

Great traditions of garden design have tended both to reflect a national identity and to show people's individual view of their relation to nature. Take, for example, the desire to control nature. The great seventeenth-century Dutch and French gardens, with their intricate formal parterres, long allées, clipped evergreens and perfect symmetry, express total control over nature, almost a desire to keep it at bay. In France they expressed royal power and were made by armies.

The creation of a small formal garden seems to appeal to those who like order, pattern and balance. Partly this is a matter of fashion (and formal garden design is certainly enjoying a revival) but it is also a matter of personal taste. Nothing that grows is allowed to become out of control. Strongly structured visual shapes – as in topiary – often provide a vertical element in a garden planned mainly as a horizontal pattern.

The informal garden

At the other end of the scale are people to whom the essence of nature is that it is uncontrolled. The idea of a wild garden often appeals to them, as does the attempt to create an enclave for wildlife in an urban world. In Britain the reaction against Victorian formality in bedding designs led by William Robinson and Gertrude Jekyll in the early twentieth century created a new, softer tradition. Robinson was not against formality close

The essence of the cottage garden is that it is unplanned, a happy profusion of plants allowed to self-seed and where vegetables, herbs and flowers for cutting can co-exist.

to the house, but allowed greater informality as one progressed through the garden away from the house towards the wilderness beyond.

Informal gardens are often called romantic, and are frequently created by great plantsmen and women. There is a greater sense of the individuality of the plant, its shape, habit and the delight it can give in being itself. In this tradition the greatest praise is given to the gardener who can create a garden that just hovers at the boundary of being out of control. Certain plants are allowed to self-seed more or less at will and the garden evolves with the minimum of interference from the hand of the gardener. This is difficult to achieve successfully but can often give wonderful results by fortuitously good plant combinations. This sort of garden mimics many of our so-called 'wild' landscapes, which are, in fact, the product of some sort of land management.

Romantic gardens are often designed to be secret and private, a special place to commune with nature undisturbed. In a large garden such places can be created by dividing the space into a series of compartments by hedges or walls, so-called 'garden rooms'. These gardens can delight by their sense of surprise as you pass from one enclosure to the next. They can express the degree to which you wish to be contained by your environment and are essentially inward-looking, like the monastery gardens of the Middle Ages.

Gardens designed with outward vistas are often planned by people who prefer to be unenclosed and who feel rather uncomfortably 'hemmed in' by hedges and fences. In the eighteenth century this was achieved by the 'ha-ha', a ditch which acted as a sunken fence to prevent ingress by stock or intruders but allowed the garden to appear as if it continued into the countryside. Today, also, gardens designed to incorporate a view can express your relation to the outside world, that part of space that you may see, but which lies beyond the area that you may design.

A FORMAL GARDEN

Aformal garden is one where plants are grown within a symmetrical pattern of beds and the paths obey the rules of geometry rather than the more cursive flow of nature. All the early gardens were formal because they were established for practical use: to produce crops for the kitchen, medicinal plants for 'physic' use, fruits for the table, even (as the gardens of Pompeii show) plant material for the making of garlands. The pattern of paths made for easy access (they were often quartered in design) and the beds were usually raised slightly, which made for easier cropping.

The formal garden tradition is very adaptable to modern-day use because it can be scaled down in size to fit most regular-shaped spaces. It is particularly useful in walled gardens and can fit into a section carved out of a more informal layout by hedges or fences, so forming a secret 'garden within a garden'.

How to design a small formal garden

First of all you will need to measure your site and transfer your measurements to a paper sketch plan from which your final design can be accurately drawn. The best way to do this is with a 30m landscape architect's tape. Measure a base line, that is the longest unbroken line that can be marked out on the site, and mark all your measurements against this. Existing trees and other features that you wish to retain can be accurately plotted by measuring from two points and describing intersecting arcs with a pair of compasses to mark the position exactly.

You may need to make minor adjustments to the level of the site. Insert a peg into the ground a short distance away from the level you have chosen to match, such as a doorstep. Using a wooden lath to rest on the peg and doorstep, check with a spirit level that the peg is level. Continue to measure around the site with further pegs. By measuring from these permanent levels to the existing soil level you can work out how much soil, hardcore etc. you will need to achieve a final true level. Transfer all this information to a plan drawn at 1:50 or 1:100 scale depending on the size of the garden, with a cross-section plan to show the levels.

Now experiment on a sketch plan to produce a formal design that is pleasing to your eye and has the right mix of 'hardworks' (paths etc.) and beds. Think about the pattern the beds will form (especially if the garden can be viewed from above) and how one enters and progresses around the garden. If you wish to incorporate seating, arbours, terracotta pots, statuary or other features that will affect the ground plan consider if they are to be placed symmetrically or as end features in short views within the garden. Remember to leave enough room to move into or around these features freely so that they do not cause obstruction.

Paths and permanent features

The 'hardworks' of the garden form its structure, although it is possible, especially in a formal garden, to emphasize the layout by formally clipped plants. Nevertheless, you must have a symmetrical

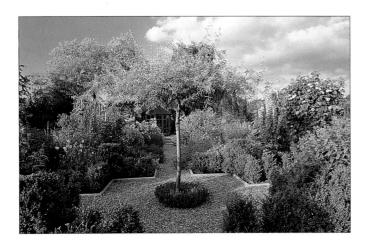

This small formal garden shows profuse herbaceous planting contained by formal bed edges and dwarf box.

arrangement, with paving materials suitable for the job. York stone, or one of the better textured modern substitutes, is an excellent but expensive choice. Any paving needs to be laid on a 7.5cm (3in) deep bed of hardcore blinded over with sand to form a level and secure base.

If you use brick you must use a weatherproof brick designed for exterior use. Brick can be laid in a variety of basket-weave or herringbone patterns that can look very attractive in a formal garden.

For a cheaper option you can use gravel, but be sure to lay it well. Lay a 7.5cm (3in) hardcore base, top this off with coarse gravel and then lay 2.5–4cm (1–1½in) of dry hoggin mix. Roll it with a heavy roller and then spread your gravel on to this. A well-laid gravel path will last for a good many years.

Planting

Plant the formal hedges in your garden next. These may be evergreen species such as box or yew, but you can also use beech which retains its browned leaves in the winter. Hornbeam makes a good deciduous hedge. Plant 60cm (2ft) apart, in a double staggered line for a thick hedge. Cut evergreen hedges between early summer and autumn, deciduous ones in the winter. For how to grow low box hedges to edge beds see page 131.

If you have little space and want to create a formal atmosphere and vertical accent, consider using trellis edging, treillage bowers as features or even low ironwork edging. All of these take up little ground horizontally but create a feeling of formal enclosure. Trellis can be attached to posts that are cemented in or, more permanently, to posts bolted on to metal stakes that do not rot.

You may also wish to copy formal features or plant varieties used in historic formal gardens, and research for this can form a fascinating pursuit for winter evenings!

When you plant the garden make sure that your selection of plants does not overwhelm the formal design by its lushness. Part of the pleasure of small formal gardens is their structure, so make sure the planting complements rather than obscures it.

VILLANDRY

The greatest flowering of the formal tradition was undoubtedly in seventeenth-century France. This was formality on a grand scale but has nevertheless inspired many scaled-down imitations in twentieth-century gardening. For example, many elements from the vegetable garden or 'potager' at Villandry in the Loire Valley can be adapted to the modern vegetable plot. The potager at Villandry contains nine squares laid out as a large parterre, edged with boxwood and with each square enclosed by a low trellis along which are trained espalier apples and pears. Vertical accent is given by standard roses (said to symbolize monks cultivating the garden) and by trellis bowers of climbing roses at major intersections. The view from the roof of the château is of a neatly patterned carpet and clearly demonstrates how formal gardens were meant to be viewed from a height. The garden is managed on a rotation, like any good vegetable garden, and ornament is introduced by sections used for low flowering plants and by the use of colourful vegetables such as ruby chard and ornamental cabbages.

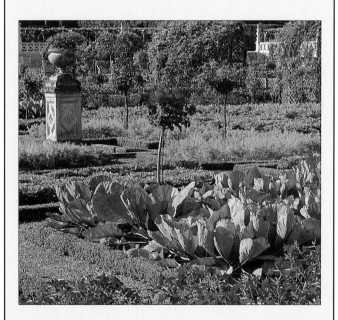

Part of the 'potager' at Villandry showing the varied greens of the produce and the floral accents.

THE ART OF TOPIARY

Topiary is the craft of forming evergreens into artificial shapes by training and clipping. It is a traditional art that was first used by the Romans but reached its heyday in gardens of the Italian Renaissance, the formal gardens of seventeenth-century France, and particularly the Netherlands, from where the tradition reached the British Isles.

Most people think of the whimsical side of the art when topiary is mentioned – the creation of peacocks, fire engines and other bizarre shapes that are quite common in cottage gardens. But there is also a structural side to topiary where hedges are used to create the boundaries in a formal garden, with individually shaped bushes of various geometric shapes acting like punctuation in a regularly structured design. This is a use of plants which resembles the way an architect uses bricks and stone, to produce the framework around the space. The tradition probably evolved from medieval knot gardens reminiscent of embroidery with their intricate designs of flowers or coloured earths bordered by low hedges.

Inspirational shapes

Few examples of historic topiary gardens remain intact though there are gardens in which topiary has obviously outgrown itself, as at Powys Castle in Wales. The best in England is at Levens Hall in Cumbria, where the designs are practically all geometric, and at Blickling Hall in Norfolk. The National Trust is growing a new garden of topiary chessmen in golden and dark green yew in the seventeenth and early eighteenth-century garden of Brickwall, Northiam, Sussex. The chessmen are being created from individual yew plants growing up within riveted iron frames to guide the gardeners in clipping the complex shapes. Another example of a chess garden can be seen at Hever Castle, in Kent.

In the USA the interest in topiary is largely confined to the east coast. There is a geometric

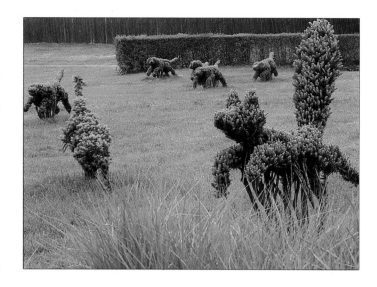

The one that got away! The fox pursued by hounds at Ladew Topiary Garden, Maryland, USA.

topiary garden at Longwood Gardens, Kennett Square, Pennsylvania, but elsewhere the emphasis is on whimsy. The most famous of these gardens are Green Animals at Portsmouth, Rhode Island, and the Ladew Topiary Garden in Maryland, where a fox hunt in full hue and cry (formed on wire frames) greets the visitor. These excesses have been copied from English and Dutch examples and remind one of the satirical inventory written by Alexander Pope at the beginning of the eighteenth century in arguing for a return to a more natural style of gardening:

Adam and Eve in yew: Adam a little shattered by the fall of the Tree of Knowledge, Eve and the serpent flourishing. Noah's ark in holly: the ribs a little damaged for want of water. St. George in box: will be in a condition to strike the dragon by next April... Divers eminent modern poets in bay, somewhat blighted... .

One wonders what Pope would have have to say about the topiary figures at Disneyland!

In the twentieth century there have been several developments in topiary. Strongly structured hedges have been used to partition large gardens into more intimate formal areas or 'rooms' within the garden. There is also a use of rectilinear hedges cut to a knife-edge precision by the skill of the gardeners, which produces an almost cubist feel to the design. Fine examples of this can be seen at Castle Drogo, on the edge of Dartmoor and at Anglesey Abbey at Stow-cum-Quy, near Cambridge, where the hedges are used as a strong piece of architecture to set off the magnificent herbaceous borders.

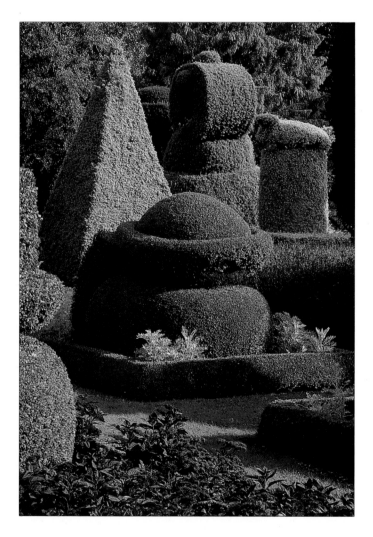

Cubism in the garden? The fine box and yew topiary at Levens Hall in Cumbria, England.

Planting and care

Currently, there is a revival in creating small formal topiary gardens in towns, and boxwood nurseries are finding a great increase in demand. The essential requirements for such a garden are a sunny, sheltered site that is level, easily accessible and large enough to accommodate a pattern of beds and topiary features. If it can be viewed from above, all the better.

Box *Buxus sempervirens* is often used to edge the beds. Plant rooted cuttings 22.5cm (9in) apart unless you want an instant effect and are able to buy three-year-old potted specimens. Topiary features can be created in box, yew or bay and you can train these yourself by trimming in late summer or you can buy ready-trimmed box cones and balls. British gardeners often buy imported specimens but they are expensive as they may have taken five to eight years to develop. Box is tolerant of any well-drained soil and is better than yew at coping with pollution in towns.

Topiary gardens require comparatively little maintenance besides a spring feed and an annual clip. If you use bay, however, you must clip with secateurs rather than shears or a hedgetrimmer and, if you use quick-growing privet, be prepared to trim your creations at least three times a year.

HOW TO TRAIN A TOPIARY SHAPE

The easiest way to create a topiary shape is to draw your design, or copy it from a book, and have it made up as a frame by a local blacksmith. If you can make your drawing actual size and place it in its final intended setting it will help you get the scale right. Ensure that the blacksmith makes the frame three-dimensional and adds a long central spike which can eventually anchor the frame in position.

Allow the plant to grow through the frame, and space out the branches and shoots to cover it. Keep the growth to the outside of the frame so that it obtains maximum light. Trim as needed. The process may take several seasons but is by far the simplest way to produce an effective shape.

A ROMANTIC GARDEN

There is a romantic element in many gardening traditions that goes back to medieval times. Here, I am using the word romantic to express an attitude to the natural world that shows reverence, wonder and nostalgia rather than the control and order that are associated with the formal garden tradition.

Romantic landscapes

In England the movement to create landscape parks out of once formal gardens, which was the hallmark of the eighteenth century, was a nostalgic attempt to recreate the classical landscapes of ancient Greece and Rome. Alexander Pope declared that 'All gardening is landscape painting', and designers such as 'Capability' Brown, Charles Bridgeman and Humphry Repton remodelled the English landscape much as if they were artists.

Great landscape gardens such as Stowe, in Buckinghamshire, and Stourhead, in Wiltshire, were created in a period when few plant species had been introduced from the botanical riches of the Far East. 'Capability' Brown (1716–83) planted with a mere handful of species to create his characteristic hilltop copses, and designed more with water and the shape of the land than with varied plant material.

The fashion for landscaping also influenced some of the formal gardens of Tuscany, where much of the formality was swept away to be replaced by lawns, as at the Villa Torrigiani, Lucca. In the USA the English landscape movement inspired Thomas Jefferson, whose garden at Monticello, started in 1769, has now been restored.

The next major boost to the romantic tradition came with the introduction of large numbers of species by the plant collectors of the late nineteenth and early twentieth centuries. A contrived wilderness became the new romantic ideal in England, much as in the USA the writers Ralph Waldo Emerson (1803–82) and Henry David Thoreau (1817–62) had celebrated the natural world and the spiritual fulfilment of living in harmony with the rural environment.

Today, romantic gardening is associated with informality in design and planting, with an emphasis on surprise and mystery and a certain joy in profuse planting. In the USA and in New Zealand cottage gardening and its use of informal perennials is especially popular. There is also great interest in the work of Gertrude Jekyll, whose long borders with great drifts of colour seem to express a lost ideal in garden beauty. Nostalgia is expressed in the rejection of new cultivars and a liking for old varieties, especially of old roses.

A garden of old roses

Any garden of old roses should be sited in full sun for the plants to thrive. Create a romantic feel by laying meandering brick or stone paths and designing bowers where you can rest on a seat and enjoy the profusion and the perfume.

Select your varieties carefully. The Alba, Centifolia, Moss and Damask roses are the finest for per-

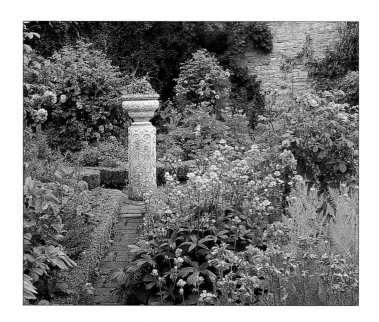

'Ispahan': a Damask once used to produce attar of roses.

fume, with the Albas having beautiful grey leaves to complement the flowers. The Moss roses have mossy, glandular growth on their buds, tempting you to touch them; so plant these close to seats in the garden where you can do so.

Most old roses only flower once in early summer, so it is as well to broaden the interest by planting some of the Portland or Bourbon roses which have two main flushes of flower, or some of the Gallicas which are virtually perpetual flowering. Specialist old-rose growers will be able to advise. Only plant the perpetual-flowering China roses (such as the delightful 'Cécile Brunner') if your garden is very warm and protected.

You will notice that all of the old roses have flowers in the white, pink and red range. This is because yellow was not introduced into rose breeding until the French started working with *Rosa foetida* in the 1870s. So it is best to choose edging plants for the rose garden from the soft colour range to suit them, such as any of the cottage pinks and *Nepeta* × *faassenii*.

SOME FAVOURITE OLD ROSES

Rose classification	Cultivar name	Height and spread	Comment
Albas	'Celestial'	1.8 × 1.2m (6 × 4ft)	Soft pink blooms, very grey foliage.
	'Maiden's Blush'	1.5 × 1.2m (5 × 4ft)	Loose habit, blush-pink flowers.
Bourbons	'Boule de Neige'	1.5 × 1.2m (5 × 4ft)	Red-tinted buds and double white flowers. Upright habit.
	'Louise Odier'	1.8 × 1.2m (5 × 4ft)	Lilac-pink flowers. Good foliage.
	'Mme Isaac Pereire'	2 × 1.5m (7 × 5ft)	Cerise-pink flowers.
Centifolias	'De Meaux'	1–1.2 × 1m (3–4 × 3ft)	Tight pink flowers. Good for small gardens.
	'Fantin Latour'	1.8 × 1.5m (6 × 5ft)	Very profuse pale pink flowers. Named for the French artist.
Damasks	'Celsiana'	1.5 × 1.2m (5 × 4ft)	Loose, blush-pink flowers.
	'Mme Hardy'	1.8 × 1.5m (6 × 5ft)	Fine white flowers.
Gallicas	'Charles de Mills'	1.5 × 1.2m (5 × 4ft)	Crimson-purple flowers.
	'Tuscany'	1.2 × 1m (4 × 3ft)	Maroon flowers.
Moss	'Common Moss'	1.2 × 1.2m (4 × 4ft)	Rounded pink blooms.
	'Shailer's White Moss'	1.2 × 1m (4 × 3ft)	White flowers, tinted pink when immature.
	'Soupert et Notting'	1–1.2 × 1m (3–4 × 3ft)	Best pink-flowered moss rose for small gardens.
Portlands	'Comte de Chambord'	1.2 × 1m (4 × 3ft)	Very profuse double pink flowers.
	'The Portland Rose'	60 × 60cm (2 × 2ft)	Crimson flowers. Excellent for restricted space.

STILL WATER: POOLS FOR CONTEMPLATION

○

Pools of water exert an irresistible fascination. Throughout the centuries and all over the world garden designers have used still water for its power to reflect. The designers of famous buildings, such as the Taj Mahal at Agra and the Palm House at Kew, constructed water features purely to mirror their outlines.

We respond to water as a life-giver and as a focal point for tranquil contemplation. Nowhere is this more true than in China where still water in a garden is used to express serenity. A flat sheet of water is also used as a complement to the vertical elements of the garden in the Chinese quest for balance in all things.

Great lakes

In eighteenth-century Britain, 'Capability' Brown designed huge lakes as part of his vision of the classic Arcadian landscape. He produced natural lakes (in fact, carefully contrived) in many of his great commissions, for example at Blenheim Palace, near Oxford, and at Chatsworth, Derbyshire. Henry Hoare's garden at Stourhead was designed around a large lake to produce delightful reflections of classical temples. Today, it is also valued for the equally lovely reflections of autumn colour from the mature trees.

In the USA a fine eighteenth-century water garden was created at Middleton Place, near Charleston, South Carolina, on the side of the Ashley River. Now restored to its former glory, it features many terraced lakes, probably inspired by the rice fields that made its owner, Henry Middleton, wealthy. At Dumbarton Oaks, near Washington, there is a lovely formal pebble garden designed to be covered by a shallow sheet of water to enrich the colour of the stones and to reflect the surrounding trees.

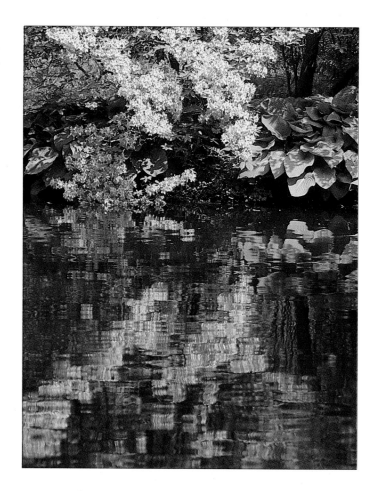

ABOVE: *Reflective water doubles the visual impact.*
RIGHT: *Dramatic leaf shapes are mirrored in still pools.*

Designing your own pool

There are obvious design features you should provide for in designing a pool. The reflections should be easily visible from the various viewpoints in the garden and the surface area should be as generous as you can afford. Aquatic plants grow extremely quickly and you may need to cull growth regularly to maintain the reflective area.

MARGINAL PLANTS TO PRODUCE REFLECTIONS

Aquatic plants can be very invasive, so you need to choose tall varieties that will cast reflections from the margins of a pool, rather than invade it. Here are some suggestions.

Common name	Botanical name	Height	Comment
Angel's Fishing Rod	*Dierama pulcherrimum*	1.2m (4ft)	Pretty, arching habit. Plant on bank.
Corkscrew Rush	*Juncus effusus* 'Spiralis'	45cm (1.5ft)	Curious twisted stems.
Dwarf Reedmace	*Typha minima*	30−75cm (1−2½ft)	Good for small pools.
Water Canna	*Thalia dealbata*	1−8m (6ft)	Needs winter protection.
Water Flag	*Iris pseudacorus*	1.5m (5ft)	Very erect habit, yellow flowers.
Water Iris	*Iris laevigata* varieties	75cm (2½ft)	Use where the Water Flag is too tall.
Zebra Sedge	*Scirpus tabernaemontani* 'Zebrinus'	1m (3ft)	Foliage banded green and white.

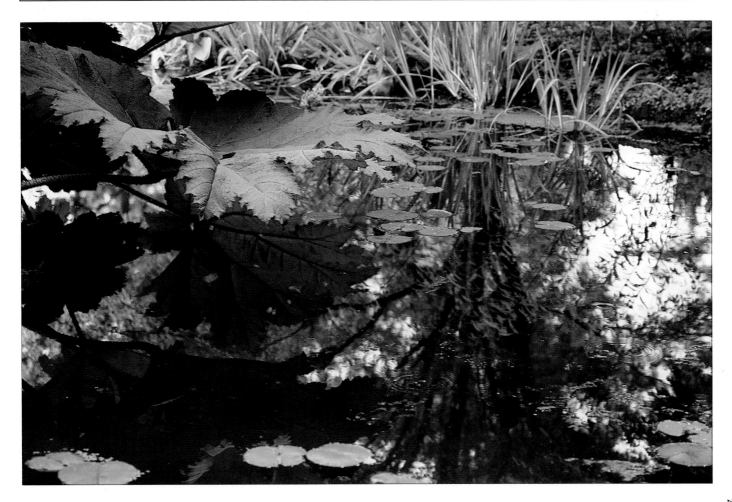

This is particularly important if you have planted water lilies as they can easily smother a pool. Remember also that pools can become dangerous when completely covered with vegetation because it is not always clear that water lies beneath rather than solid ground.

There are three main methods of creating a pool: with a butyl rubber liner, a pre-formed (usually fibreglass) liner, and concrete. The easiest method is to use a good-quality liner, especially a black liner which makes the water appear darker and more reflective. This is ideally suited to an informal design, but you can also use one to line a formal raised pool created from brickwork or concrete formwork. This type of pool may be more suitable to a small town garden or where toddlers need to be protected from falling in.

Create a pool to complement your garden: an octagon, square or some other symmetrical shape lined up with other lines in the garden is suited to a formal garden, whereas a pond with curved outlines suits an informal or wild garden. Do not obscure the edges of a formal pool with spreading plants; use erect iris or rushes placed symmetrically. Use more rampant plants around an informal pool to blend into its surroundings.

Consider the siting for the pool. It should be away from overhanging trees that will drop their leaves and pollute it. Aquatic plants need good light to grow well. Avoid placing the pool where it will create unwanted reflections.

You need still water for the cultivation of water lilies. These are best planted in tubs of unsterilized loam and then sited in the water. Choose varieties that are suited in vigour to the size of the pool and the depth of the water.

A garden that is used at night looks best if it is well lit. Pools themselves can be floodlit from above or illuminated by submerged lights, adding an extra quality to the scene. In some countries a qualified contractor must be used for this type of installation to ensure the safe use of electrical equipment near water.

The informal lake at Claude Monet's garden at Giverny in France is rich in marginal plants and soft-coloured reflections.

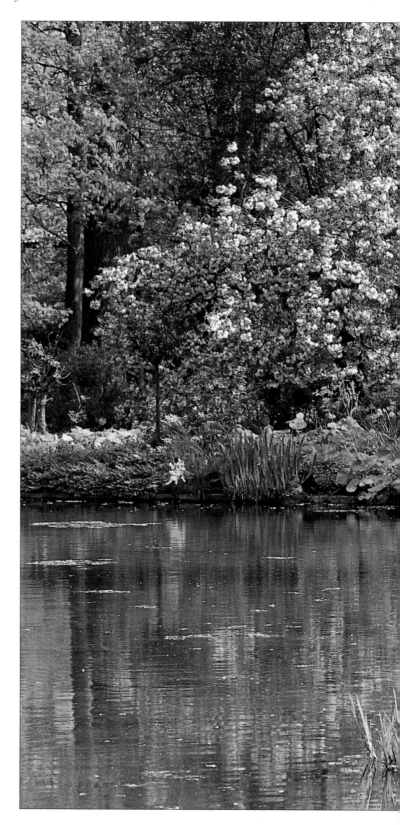

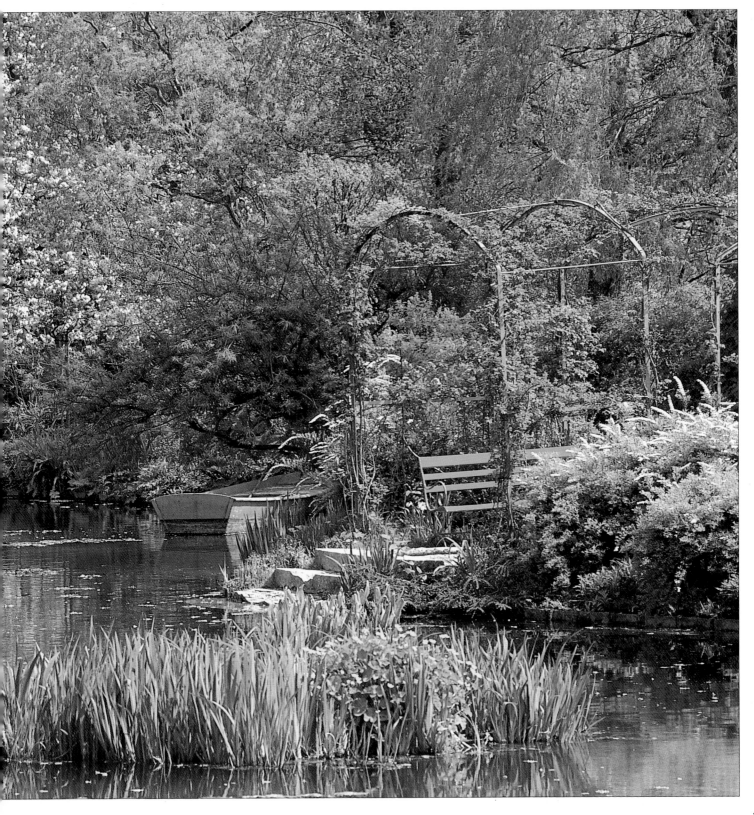

THE MYSTICAL MAZE

○

'For what the centre brings
Must obviously be
That which remains to the end
And was there from eternity'
GOETHE (1749–1832)

The tradition of building mazes is very old and seems to express a psychological need to solve puzzles and attain a goal. Psychologists recognize this as an intrinsically healing move towards wholeness – the centring of the self. How satisfying to find your way through the labyrinth with the chance to review the wrong choices made and turning points missed!

The patterns of mazes dating back to 2000 BC can be seen carved in rock in Sardinia, and somewhat later in Italy, India and Egypt. They also occur as earthworks or as patterns built on the ground with stones, and in Greek mythology the maze is the site where Theseus slays the Minotaur. These early labyrinths possessed a single path to the centre and would be used ritually to symbolize the path of life, and walked either by individuals or by community processions. There are, for example, over 400 of these ancient mazes in Scandinavia.

The early mazes usually had seven rings, a number traditionally thought to be magical, but the medieval Christian church produced a strong history of maze design with eleven rings, perhaps representing the 'true' apostles. These mazes, clearly religious and meditational in intent, were built as circles or octagons into the floor design of the naves of many of the cathedrals in northern France, including Amiens. The best, and oldest, example is in blue and white marble in Chartres cathedral (AD 1235). Known as the 'Path to Jerusalem', it clearly symbolizes the Christian crusades and the attempt to reach Jerusalem and salvation. Penitents may have followed the path of the maze on their knees as was common practice in medieval Europe. The tradition of using coloured stone to mark out these patterns is often seen in modern churches, though usually in the sanctuary rather than the nave. They point to the continuing spiritual value of mazes wherever they are created.

Garden mazes

The tradition of mazes for ritual and religious use was taken into gardens in the form of turf mazes cut into the grass and intended for meditation or sometimes for penance. In Britain, the tradition seems to be linked with Norse settlement and one can still be seen at Dalby, North Yorkshire. The largest, at 35 metres (96ft) across, is on the common at Saffron Walden in Essex. In gardens, turf mazes exist at Somerton, Oxfordshire, and at

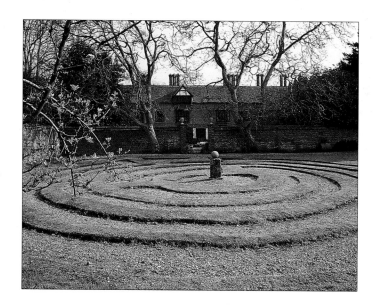

Turf mazes were intended for processional meditation. This modern maze was laid to a sixteenth-century design.

Chenies Manor in Buckinghamshire.

Secular mazes were built in the gardens of royalty and the wealthy as places of amusement. These were usually hedge puzzle mazes made by growing yew or cypress. The earliest were in France, Spain and Italy in the late seventeenth and early eighteenth centuries. In the Netherlands one was built between 1686 and 1695 for the splendid palace of William and Mary at Het Loo. The world-famous Hampton Court maze was built by George London and Henry Wise between 1689 and 1696. Its design was copied many times during the 'maze craze' of the late nineteenth century in the USA and Britain when many were laid out in public parks, and in the Governor's Palace maze, Williamsburg, Virginia, in 1935. The hedges in these were all taller than the height of a man, so making the puzzle more difficult to solve. They sometimes contained some high point from which an overview of the puzzle could be obtained as, for example, in the huge maze at Longleat House, Wiltshire, designed in 1978. The circular maze at Stra, near Venice, built in 1720, contained a tower at its centre with a double spiral staircase, perhaps an uncanny portent of the double helix structure of molecules discovered to be at the centre of life!

The designs of mazes sited near great houses were usually formal, like parterres, and were rectangular or square, as at Hatfield House, Hertfordshire, laid out in the 1980s. There are fewer informal mazes but there is an interesting one in laurel at Glendurgan, Cornwall (1833). At Leeds Castle, Kent, there is an inspirational maze, built in 1988, that leads the visitor to an underground grotto as if on a journey through the Underworld. Several recent mazes have been built like the imprint of a footprint, as if a giant had walked upon the Earth.

Today, new mazes are usually sited in a garden or a park, which emphasizes their recreational role. Garden hedge mazes are usually planted in slow-growing evergreens such as yew, cypress, holly or elaeagnus, which require clipping once a year. Turf mazes are inexpensive to install but difficult to maintain due to wear and tear unless the trodden route is made of gravel, brick or paving between the turf.

Mazes do not have to be made out of living plants. They can be created on the flat, in brick with water between, or with verticals in wood (a design that is particularly popular in Japan and in New Zealand).

One maze designer has estimated that in the 1980s the number of mazes available for public access more than doubled. There is no doubt that the universal mystical appeal of these garden puzzles continues to fascinate, and a small maze in your own garden might become quite a talking point among your guests!

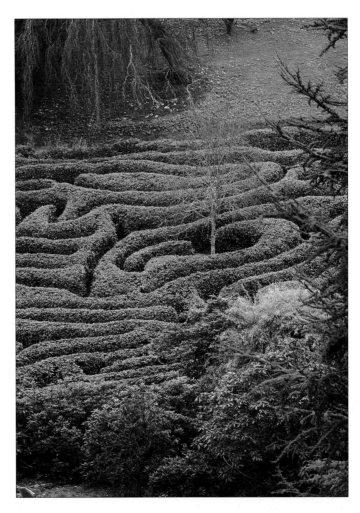

The laurel maze at Glendurgan, Cornwall, England, is unusual in being informal as well as being planted on a slope.

SCULPTURE IN THE GARDEN

Sculpture has been a traditional element in the design of a good garden since Roman times, and it has always had a wide variety of functions. On large estates it has often expressed the power and wealth of the owner. In many domestic gardens, however, sculpted material has frequently been placed for practical purposes; for example, assisting with telling the time or covering a wellhead.

Any garden, except the very smallest, can make use of sculpture in creating a pleasing structure to the design or in reinforcing the overall layout. A well-sited item can act as a focal point or mark a change in direction, almost leading you through the construction of the garden rather like punctuation in a sentence. Paired sculptures (for example, either side of the entrance) can produce a pleasing sense of balance. Almost without noticing you are likely to feel 'contained' by such an arrangement; if an item is missing or not quite the same size, the effect can be disturbing.

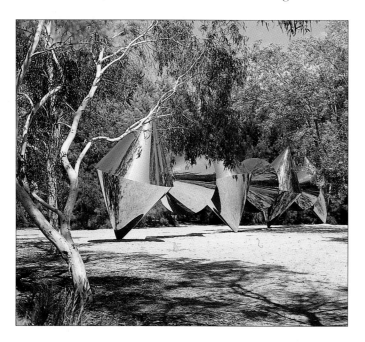

Stainless steel amid the heat and sand in Canberra, Australia.

Figurative sculpture also introduces the human element into the natural scene. On the other hand, some modern abstract sculpture with hard linear outlines oddly looks very effective against a background of plants, perhaps because of the obvious contrast with natural forms. Both types of sculpture can provide objects of contemplation and, if well sited, can be used to cast attractive shadows on a lawn, thus increasing their three-dimensional effect. They perform the essential function of all art, to surprise and to disturb as well as to please.

Buying and placing items

One of the first considerations in your mind should be matching the age and style of your sculpture with the period of your garden. Appropriateness is the key. Next, consider scale. This is the most difficult consideration to get right; your chosen item must be the right scale for its immediate surroundings. If it is too small it will look lost; if too large it will dominate and appear ridiculous. If necessary, make a template or a sketch on a board to see what size of item fits the position you have in mind and take these dimensions with you to the salerooms!

To get some ideas about the placement of sculpture, try visiting gardens where there are good collections. Anglesey Abbey, at Stow-cum-Quy near Cambridge, England, has a superb collection of classical bronze, lead and stone statuary which is very well placed. Chiswick House in London also has an impressive array. Most of the great Italian gardens, such as the Villa Aldobrandini at Frascati, have excellent examples of niche statuary and so do many in France. Gardens incorporating modern sculpture include the gardens of the Art Museum in Canberra, Australia, the Carl Milles Garden in Stockholm and the Abby Aldrich Rockefeller Sculpture Garden at the Museum of Modern Art in New York.

Also consider the background you are able to

provide. Pale stone items look good against dark-leaved hedges such as yew. Perhaps you have a view through a gate that can frame a sculpture placed as you approach the gate. If you are planning a wall, you may be able to 'design in' a niche for an object, or cut out an opening in a hedge to see a sculpture through it and framed by it.

Materials

When you are thinking about buying statuary consider the expense of original items against that of reconstructed stone copies and replicas. If you are attracted to terracotta, which is particularly popular in Tuscan gardens, then do make sure that what you buy is frostproof. Then you can leave it out in winter without it cracking or flaking. Sculpture in the garden does not need to be in the conventional materials of stone, bronze, lead or terracotta. It can be made in slate or even in wicker. In the last decade wicker figures have become popular at some of the major flower shows. Wicker needs special treatment (see page 142). If you have a wild garden you can use wicker and other wood products rather in the way that they have been used in some of the 'sculpture trails' laid out in forest environments. Places to see them are Grizedale Sculpture Park in Cumbria, England, and the Landmark Visitors' Centre, Carrbridge, Scotland.

Lighting sculpture

The art of using sculpture in the garden is its correct placement. You can also use natural light to emphasize your sculpture, siting it where sunbeams will alight. If you use the garden at night, consider the use of lighting to bring out the full dramatic potential of a piece. Floodlighting will create strong shadows and concealed uplighting can focus the eye upon an object.

If you have still water in the garden, placing a statue near it (or in it) will obviously double the height and effect by the reflection, as in a mirror. The Japanese combine this idea with lighting effects, designing special stone lanterns intended to hold candles which project over the water to create a double image of the flickering light.

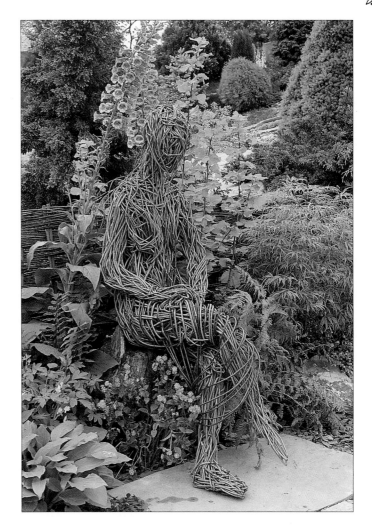

Wicker is the least durable of sculptural materials, but is highly effective in woodland settings and against hurdle fencing.

Interactive sculpture

Just as, over the years, myriad pairs of young hands have polished the ears of the bronze rabbits around the base of the sculpture of Peter Pan in Kensington Gardens, London, many sculptures cry out to be touched. Bronze and lead have wonderful textures and give a strong tactile pleasure. The smooth curves of Henry Moore pieces invite caresses. In your own garden it is important to place tactile pieces where they can be touched without plants being disturbed or blocking access.

If the joy of the piece is more visual, then place it where it can be seen from all sides against the sky. Some of the recent work in sculpture parks invites the audience to participate. For example, at Grizedale some of the wooden sculptures are like odd buildings which the public can enter to rearrange the contents so the sculpture is never the same.

Trompe-l'oeil

If you have very little space on the ground but are surrounded by walls (as in a town courtyard garden) you can make use of 'tricks of the eye' to increase the sense of space. Often this is done by fixing trellis ('treillage') specially designed with trick perspective on to the wall. Mirrors can also be used behind sculpted figures to increase their three-dimensional effect. 'Sculpture' can be painted on to wood, then aged and chipped, to appear authentic from a little distance. This is difficult to do well and it is best to employ a firm skilled in this sort of work.

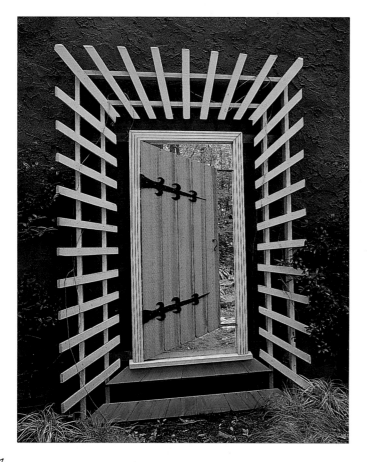

| CARING FOR STATUARY AND OTHER SCULPTURE |

Stone
Sandstone and limestone are the stone materials with the longest life, but limestone will inevitably degrade over the decades in a city environment through the effect of acid pollutants in the air.

You can age stone by brushing it with a liquid manure mix; this will encourage moss growth.

Lead
Lead needs no special care and will naturally take on a soft grey bloom. It looks especially good next to pink flowers and silver-leaved plants.

Bronze
Bronze can be left natural or waxed to enrich the patina.

Hardwood
Leave hardwood to weather to a grey appearance or oil it yearly to keep the original colour.

You can achieve an aged appearance quickly by using wood bleach.

Wicker
Treat annually with a wood preservative to prolong the life of wicker and preserve its colour.

Resin and fibreglass
Clean these synthetic materials with detergent as needed.

Terracotta
Terracotta urns that are planted are often discoloured by the leaching out of fertilizer salts that leave a whitish deposit. These can be cleaned off using a mild acid such as kettle descaler, but it is easier to avoid the problem by painting the inside of the urn with a non-toxic sealant paint before planting it up.

LEFT: Trompe l'oeil: *a door or not a door?*
RIGHT: *Garden sculpture should surprise. 'Seated girl' by Bernard Sindell.*

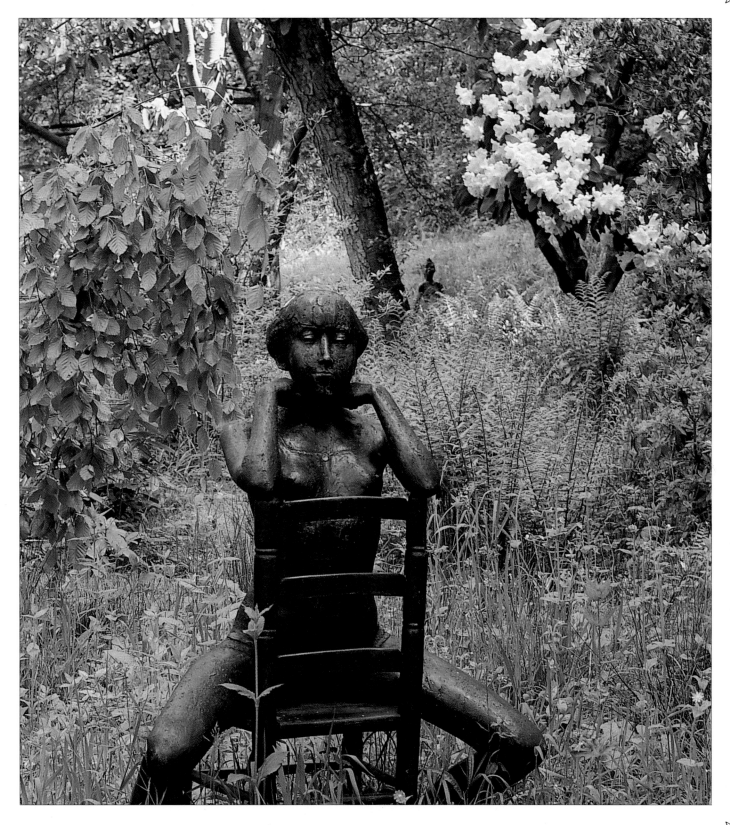

THE URBAN WILDLIFE GARDEN

○

It is a strange paradox that whereas people used to go into the countryside to seek contact and observe wildlife, modern farming practices have forced wildlife itself into cities. The urban garden can become a refuge for all sorts of birds, mammals and invertebrates and this contact with nature can be enjoyed first hand by anyone with a small patch of land and some basic hints on how to encourage living creatures.

If you consider the area covered by domestic gardens, good practices here could form the basis of a huge 'nature reserve' where wildlife has a sanctuary against pesticide use and habitat loss. There are many ways you can encourage creatures to visit (for example, providing food and nest boxes for birds) but it is much more exciting to try and recreate a small area of a natural habitat. This means understanding something of ecology and the various food chains necessary to make the habitat fully functional.

Planning a wildlife garden

There are a number of elements necessary to a wildlife garden for it to be ecologically successful: a nectar border to attract butterflies and moths; a pond, with an area for moisture-loving plants next to it; a meadow or flowery bank (preferably edged with a hedge); and an area representative of the edge of a woodland, a very diverse and species-rich environment.

The nectar border is the element closest to familiar garden design and you should site this in a sunny, sheltered position preferably close to, and easily viewed from, the house. Select plants from the species listed in the table on page 145.

A pond can be created using a liner (see page 136), and you can extend the liner (punctured in a few places) under an adjacent bed to create an area with impeded drainage. This makes an excellent wetland habitat that you can plant with species such as the Marsh Marigold *Caltha palustris*, Meadowsweet *Filipendula ulmaria*, Monkey flower

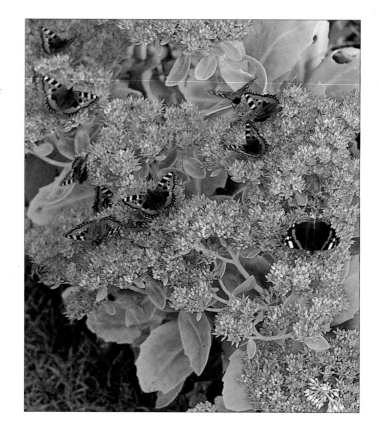

Sedum spectabile is one of the best autumn-flowering perennials to attract tortoiseshell butterflies.

Mimulus guttatus, Purple Loosestrife *Lythrum salicaria*, Yellow Flag *Iris pseudacorus* and the aquatic Forget-me-Not *Myosotis scorpioides*, all of which are very colourful as well as attractive to insects.

Many people like the idea of wildflower gardening while at the same time finding a lawn too much to manage. Providing your soil is of fairly low fertility you can sow a wildflower meadow with seed mixtures specially prepared for this, or even of specially selected cornfield weeds. This would normally need to be mown once in late summer, but you can provide access by regularly mowing an informal path through it weekly.

Hedgerow habitats have been decimated by the drive for agricultural efficiency. You can imitate a hedgerow environment by planting a mixed hedge of native species, rather than the ubiquitous privet or Leyland Cypress. In Britain plant species such as Blackthorn, Sea Buckthorn, Dogwood, Elder, Hawthorn, Hazel and Dog Rose. These provide berries and fruits for wildlife. Trim the hedge in winter when in least use by birds and mammals.

Towards the edge of your garden you might like to create an area to imitate a woodland edge. Use native trees and shrubs to provide shade, and import logs and stumps or make a woodpile that can rot and provide habitats for insects and invertebrates. Once an area is established you can underplant it with Bluebells, Wood Anemones, Herb Paris and other native flowers of the forest floor. Use your woodland area to site nestboxes and you will probably find birds will use them if you have encouraged the provision of food for them by your management of the rest of the garden. You can also encourage hedgehogs (wonderful destroyers of slugs) by leaving a box filled with straw in a wooded area of the garden. Hedgehogs are territorial and if one 'adopts' you, nothing is nicer than feeding it pet food at night and feeling honoured by the visits! This contact with nature can be a real refuge from the artificiality of much urban living.

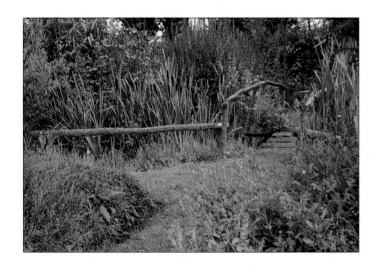

A good wildlife garden should contain a pond and wetland habitat, a rough-mown flowery bank and a woodland edge.

PLANTS TO ENCOURAGE BUTTERFLIES AND OTHER INSECTS

Botanical name/common name

Agrostemma githago Corncockle	A
Buddleja davidii varieties Butterfly bushes	S
Caryopteris × *clandonensis*	S
Ceanothus varieties Californian Lilacs	S
Centaurea cyanus Cornflower	A
Dipsacus fullonum Teasel	B
Eupatorium cannabinum Hemp Agrimony	P
Hebe species and cultivars	S
Heliotropium cultivars Heliotrope	A
Hyssopus officinalis Hyssop	S
Lavandula (all varieties)	S
Lonicera periclymenum Honeysuckle	C
Reseda odorata Mignonette	A
Saponaria officinalis Soapwort	P
Sedum (Hylotelephium) spectabile	P
Spiraea japonica 'Bumalda'	S
Thymus varieties Thyme	P
Verbena bonariensis Verbena	P
Viburnum tinus	S

PLANTS THAT PROVIDE FOOD FOR BIRDS

Botanical name/common name

Aster novi-belgii Michaelmas Daisies	P
Berberis × *stenophylla* Barberry	S
Cornus sanguinea Dogwood	S
Cosmos species	A/P
Cotoneaster horizontalis	S
Elaeagnus angustifolia	S
Euonymus europaeus Spindle	S
Helianthus annuus Sunflower	A
Ilex aquifolium Holly	S/T
Lonicera periclymenum Honeysuckle	C
Malus 'John Downie' Crab Apple	T
Oenothera biennis Evening Primrose	B
Prunus padus Bird Cherry	T
Pyracantha 'Mohave' Firethorn	S
Sambucus nigra Elder	S/T
Sorbus aucuparia Rowan	T
Taxus baccata Yew	T
Viburnum opulus Guelder Rose	S

KEY:

A Annual; B Biennial; C Climber; P Perennial; S Shrub; T Tree.

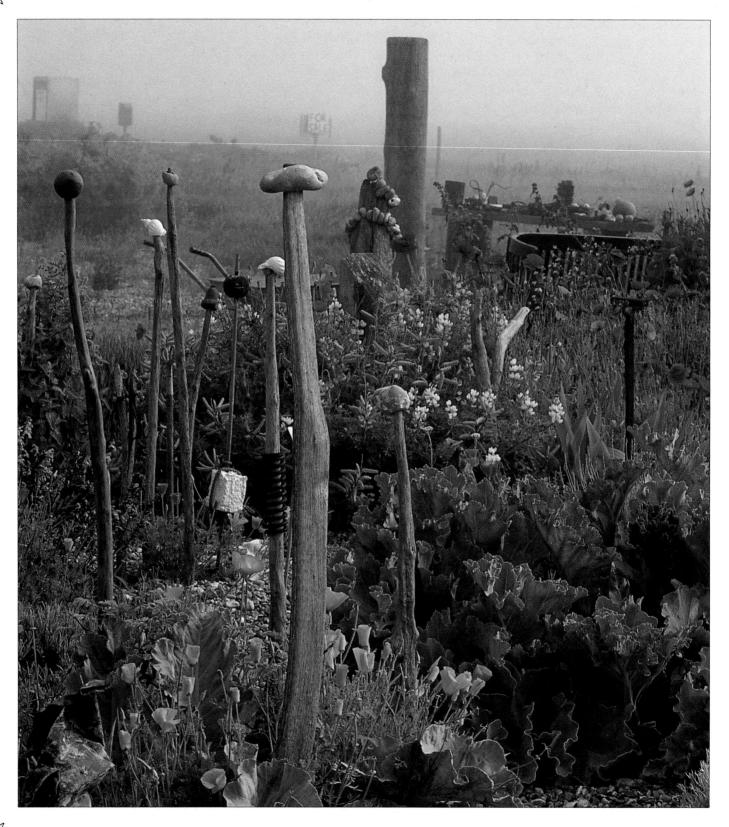

A PLACE FOR SELF-EXPRESSION

○

If you are limited to a mundane job, the garden is often the only place where you can express yourself freely and creatively. It allows you to develop aspects of your personality that may be denied elsewhere. For example, in the nineteenth century there was a great tradition among the miners of Nottinghamshire, England, in growing and showing auriculas and laced pinks. This was exacting and meticulous work, requiring patience and pride, yet different from their shifts underground. Like the Welsh tradition of growing championship leeks, it also allowed people to socialize, to compete and to excel. For many, the garden was a place of absorbing interest totally different from their workaday lives and a place of privacy and healing recreation.

Choosing the unusual

One of the commonest ways of demonstrating individuality in your garden is via topiary (see page 130). You can proclaim your interests to your neighbours in privet battleships or yew submarines. A front garden can be populated with topiary peacocks, owls, eagles or whatever takes your fancy. There is also a tradition of creating miniature worlds complete with villages, livestock and people. Shell gardens are often found at homes by the sea. Here the element of horticulture is almost negligible, the absorption being in the making of models, and the garden is just the space used to do so.

At Crystal Palace Park in South London there is a landscape complete with lifesize model dinosaurs emerging from the undergrowth, so that you can imagine yourself back in that prehistoric era. The Victorians delighted in such ideas, just as in eighteenth-century England there was a fad for creating classic landscapes, complete with hermits employed to inhabit rustic grottoes. The

Bizarre or self-expressive? The shingle garden of the film director Derek Jarman on the bleak Kent coast.

space of the garden is, and always was, the gardener's space to create the 'world as wanted', even though to others it might seem the height of bad taste. Complete models of Stonehenge in stone or flint might not seem like everyone's idea of an appropriate centrepiece for a front garden, but they may be the pride and joy of the owner.

Grand ideas

Gardens are also places where the gardener can make political statements, proclaiming the national flag in bedding or the colours of a political party in a ribbon border. The Victorians produced some extraordinary plant confections in their parks, creating models of crowns and animals on frames in dwarf bedding. This tradition remains today only at large shows such as the Chelsea Flower Show, England, or in well-funded establishments such as Longwood Gardens in Pennsylvania, USA.

Some of the more bizarre ideas I have encountered recently include a garden of summer bedding entirely in black and white, and a flat maze created from brilliantly coloured plastic looking rather like a large executive puzzle.

By tradition great estates have sometimes been created in a way which literally remodels the world. In the eighteenth century 'Capability' Brown used vast numbers of workmen to flatten hills and dig out lakes to create the views he wanted in his garden designs. In gardens such as Biddulph Grange in Staffordshire, the Victorians created a world within a world, with gardens representing ancient Egypt and China. This is paralleled today by Sir Geoffrey Jellicoe's plans for the Moody Gardens, a vast 'garden of gardens' on the coast of the Gulf of Mexico in which every national style of garden will be recreated from classical times to the present. This is creating on a large scale what many of us do in a far smaller area, creating a patch that is our own and in a style that gives us pleasure and recreation.

A JAPANESE GARDEN

○

For the Japanese, gardens have always represented a strongly religious world view that is totally different from that of the West. Whereas the tradition of a 'lost paradise' is at the heart of landscape design in Christian and Arabic traditions, the strong Shinto and Taoist beliefs in Japan stress unity with nature through the balancing of contradictory elements and the attainment of a blissful state. Their gardens are thus more contemplative, meditative and strongly symbolic or allegorical. The ideas of yin (the still, female element in the creation) and of yang (the moving principle, the male) are as important here as they are in Chinese medicine (see page 35).

Creating your own Japanese garden

Water and stone are the two essential features in any Japanese garden but it is the skill of composition that makes it truly Japanese. Moving water, a yang force, must balance with areas of reflective still water representing the yin. This is not difficult to achieve with waterfalls, fountains and pools (some construction details are given on pages 100 and 136). Make use of weathered stone to represent mountains, and areas of sand and cobbles to represent softer hill and vale, placing them asymmetrically so that the design is as naturalistic as possible.

Your plant selection should stress evergreens, especially dwarf conifers. If you use some of the fine Japanese maples for autumn colour, use them in partial shade and plant moss beneath them. Do not mass flowers together; the Japanese plant them with restraint and as simple individual elements to enhance the overall design. Use traditional Japanese materials such as split bamboo for fencing to give an authentic style. Incorporating a semi-shaded area, where you can site bonsai to use as objects of contemplation that express the forces of nature, also makes an interesting and attractive feature.

A good Japanese garden can be constructed in quite a small space, such as a courtyard, or even a tiny area if you restrict yourself to growing bonsai. However, if you wish to create a sizeable garden, plan to include walks and small pavilions in the Japanese manner. If you can visit Japan for inspiration, go to the restored Golden Pavilion and the Silver Pavilion in Kyoto to get some ideas about garden architecture. The Katsura Imperial Palace, also in Kyoto, is a good example of a meditative garden where walks were designed to express the soul's journey through the world, much as in the West people would walk around contemplative mazes or labyrinths (see page 138). Fine examples of Japanese gardens created far from their homeland can be seen in San Francisco and in Brooklyn Botanic Gardens, New York.

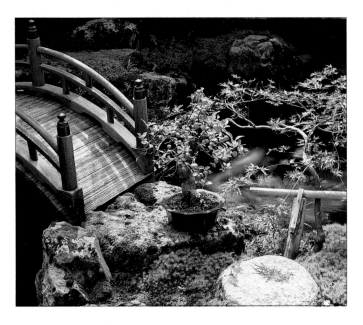

ABOVE: *Bonsai, bridges and bamboo: important elements in the design of any Japanese garden, as are acers and asymmetry.*

RIGHT: *A Zen Buddhist garden is representative of the forces of nature. Stone symbolizes the 'male and female principles' while 'gardening' becomes raking and meticulous leaf-picking. This one is unusual in not being sited within a courtyard.*

A ZEN GARDEN OF CONTEMPLATION

The so-called dry gardens of Zen Buddhism were originally designed for silent contemplation by monks and made little use of plants. Traditionally these gardens were walled and featured sand raked into designs to represent flowing water, with stones placed to represent mountains. The 'gardening' or raking of stones or large pebbles was an act of worship and the tea ceremonies the monks went through were designed to refresh them and keep them awake during their long hours of meditation.

If you wish to create such a garden you will need a regular-shaped area well away from overhanging deciduous trees, and the garden will need to be bordered, either by walls or bamboo fencing. Lay the area of stone rather like a path with a 7.5cm (3in) depth of hardcore, blinded over with gravel and with the stone on top. This should prevent weeds emerging to spoil the design.

A Zen garden can be used for peaceful meditation; it is also a garden that needs minimum attention and may well suit a busy person. Do not design one, however, if you like the business of growing plants, since the concept provides little opportunity!

Good Zen gardens can be seen in Japan at the Daisen monastery and at Ryōan-ji in the Daiju-in monastery, both in Kyoto. In the USA there is a large one in the Huntingdon Botanic Gardens, north of Los Angeles, California, and one has recently been built in the courtyard of the herbarium at the Royal Botanic Gardens, Kew, in England.

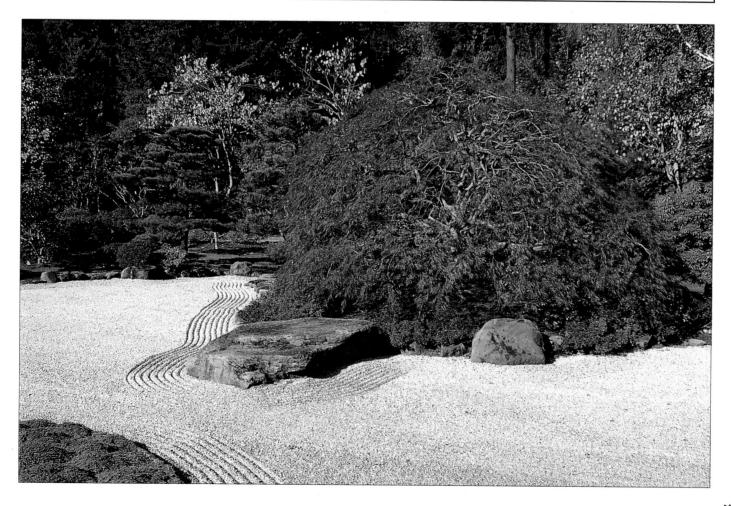

A TOWN MEDITERRANEAN GARDEN

Those who know the Mediterranean area appreciate the joy that can be found in having a small town courtyard brimming with colourful and fragrant plants that remind you of that region.

The Mediterranean climate is one of a dry, hot summer followed by a cool, fairly moist winter. Mediterranean climates can be found in all the countries bordering that sea, and also in California, Chile, South Africa and south-west Australia.

Many town gardens in southern Britain contain a microclimate that is close to that of the Mediterranean because of the heat a city generates. This warmth is increased if the garden is walled, the walls absorbing the sun's warmth by day and releasing it by night. The Chelsea Physic Garden is a perfect example of this and on a morning when the rest of the garden is frozen a one metre (3ft) area at the foot of each wall remains completely free of frost. In the garden we can grow olives, pomegranates and other tender plants that would not survive outside.

Designing a Mediterranean garden

If you have a small courtyard you may wish to lay quarry tiles or flagstones, or even insert small pebbles in the sort of intricate designs favoured in Italian and Moorish gardens. Using glazed tiles in wall niches or behind seats gives a Spanish or Portuguese atmosphere, as will the use of statuary and small fountains. Carefully placed terracotta urns appropriately planted give a Tuscan feel; try planting with small trailers such as the blue *Convolvulus sabatius*, the pink *C. althaeoides* or the startling scarlet *Lotus berthelotii*.

The plants you choose need to reflect the fact that the Mediterranean is rich in evergreens, in colourful annuals and in bulbous plants. You may also wish to include one of the hardier palms. If you have a conservatory you can grow a variety of tender shrubs in tubs (even *Citrus*) which you then bring in for winter.

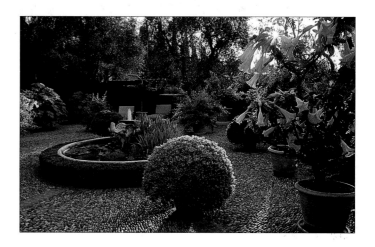

A Mediterranean courtyard in the evening. The intricate pebble paving and handsome terracottas set the scene.

Always make full use of your wall space for tender climbers and fill in at the base of sunny walls with bulbs that enjoy being baked by the sun in summer. Fill your terracotta pots with tender perennials for strong summer colour, but be prepared to replace them yearly or take cuttings to preserve them indoors over winter.

Specimen plants

You can make features of some really dramatic plants in sizeable terracotta or wooden tubs. Try using the various varieties of Angel's Trumpets (*Brugmansia*). The Coral Tree *Erythrina crista-galli* has dark red, waxy flowers in upright spikes. You can keep this for years if you regularly cut the shrub hard back in spring; it will then flower on the tips of the new growth in late summer. The Bird of Paradise *Strelitzia reginae* also has handsome leaves, but far more spectacular flowers that last for weeks both on the plant and when cut for display in vases. Remember that strelitzias need to be pot bound to flower well and that all these plants require some winter protection to survive to give you a further Mediterranean effect during the following summer months.

PLANTS FOR MEDITERRANEAN GARDENS

Here are a number of Mediterranean plants of varying sizes to give brightly coloured blooms, lush greenery and fragrance to your garden.

Botanical name/ Common name	Maximum height and spread	Comment
TREES		
c *Cercis siliquastrum* Judas Tree	4.5 × 3m (15 × 10ft)	Pretty pink flowers on the bare branches in spring.
Cupressus sempervirens 'Stricta' Italian Cypress	7.5 × 0.75m (25 × 2½ft)	Unmistakable signature of the Italian countryside.
c *Olea europaea* Olive	4.5 × 3m (15 × 10ft)	Lovely grey foliage. May fruit in very warm gardens.
c *Chamaerops humilis* European Fan Palm	1.5 × 2.5m (5 × 8ft)	Good where a shortish palm is needed.
c *Trachycarpus fortunei* Chusan Palm	7.5 × 2.5m (20 × 8ft)	Produces a stately fibre-covered trunk.
SHRUBS		
Acacia dealbata Mimosa	9 × 6m (27 × 18ft)	Lovely silver foliage and yellow flowers.
c *Albizzia julibrissin* Pink Siris Tree	6 × 6m (18 × 18ft)	Fine foliage and long-stamened pink flowers.
c *Beschorneria yuccoides*	3 × 1.8m (10 × 6ft)	A spectacular pink flower spike.
c *Ceanothus* 'Concha'	3 × 3m (10 × 10ft)	Produces extremely dark blue flowers in late spring.
c *Clianthus puniceus* Lobster's Claw	1.8 × 1.8m (6 × 6ft)	Dramatic claw-shaped flowers, usually red or pink.
c *Euphorbia mellifera*	1 × 1m (3 × 3ft)	Forms a perfect dome. Honey-scented flowers.
c *Melianthus major*	2.5 × 3m (8 × 10ft)	Lovely grey leaves, brownish-red flowers.
c *Nerium oleander*	3 × 3m (10 × 10ft)	Varieties in pink, apricot, salmon, red and white.
c* *Plumbago auriculata*	2 × 1.5m (6 × 5ft)	The purest of sky-blue flowers.
c *Punica granatum* Pomegranate (and dwarf form 'Nana')	3 × 2m (10 × 7ft) 1 × 1m (3 × 3ft)	Scarlet flowers.
c *Romneya coulteri* Tree Poppy	1.2 × 1.2m (4 × 4ft)	Grey leaves, huge white flowers.
CLIMBERS		
c *Rosa banksiae* var. *normalis* 'Lutea' Banksian Rose	7.5 × 4m (25 × 13ft)	Profuse sprays of tiny yellow flowers.
c *Trachelospermum jasminoides*	6 × 3m (20 × 10ft)	Deliciously scented.
PERENNIALS		
c* *Anthemis tinctoria*	0.75 × 0.45m (2½ × 1½ft)	Yellow daisy flowers.
c* *Argyranthemum* cultivars	0.75 × 0.45m (2½ × 1½ft)	Daisy-like flowers in a wide variety of colours.
c* *Gazania* hybrids	20–30 × 30cm (8–12 × 12in)	Striking bi-colour daisy flowers.
BULBS		
c *Amaryllis belladonna*	60 × 30cm (2 × 1ft)	Pink flowers on naked stems in autumn.
c *Scilla peruviana*	30 × 23cm (1ft × 9in)	Dense heads of blue flowers in late spring.

KEY

c Can be seen growing in the Chelsea Physic Garden, a 'Mediterranean'-type garden in central London.

* Likely not to survive winters outdoors; take cuttings in summer to perpetuate over winter under glass.

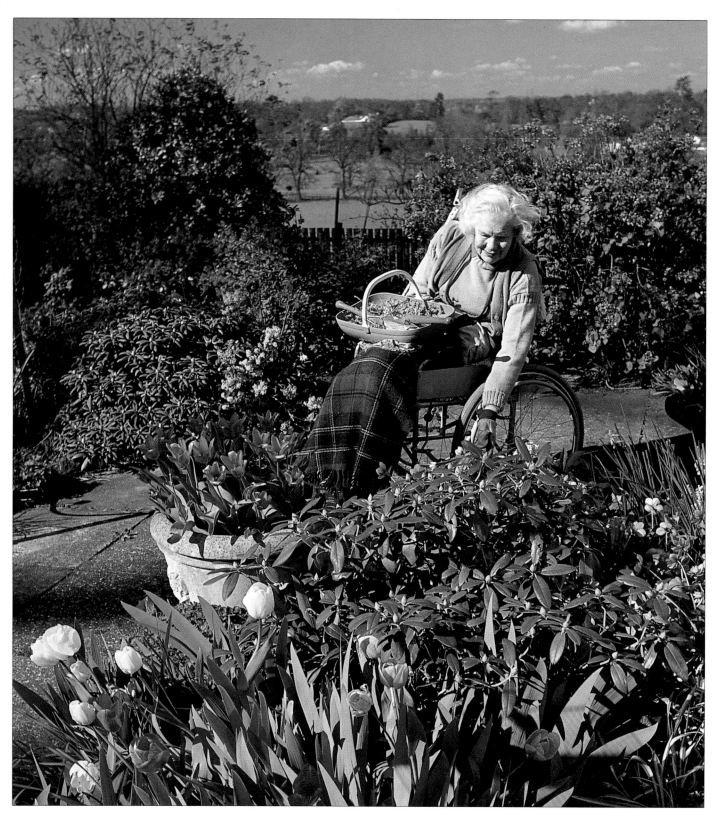

THE THERAPY OF GARDENING

Many people enjoy gardening as a therapeutic activity although they may not be consciously aware of the benefits to them. Just as 'art therapy' is recommended by therapists specializing in rehabilitation, so gardening has been adapted by these professionals as a healing 'occupational therapy'.

There must be something about the cycles of growth and change that is helpful in the treatment of the mentally ill and something also that appeals to mentally handicapped children and adults. Dealing with plants is getting back to basics; gardening involves us in the needs of plants and their responses to us can produce tremendous pleasure, particularly in those who feel isolated.

Gardening is also used as physical therapy to develop dexterity in the recovery from injury, and a great number of the tools developed to help in this area are useful to the disabled in the general community who wish to enjoy gardening. They are also helpful for the great mass of us who want to garden in retirement and need aids to help with the various health problems that limit us in age. Lifelong gardeners do not give up gardening easily and will go to great lengths to keep going!

Making access easy

For the disabled and elderly gardener alike the problems a garden can pose mainly involve access, but there are many ways these can be solved with a bit of pre-planning and investment. For example, can you eliminate steps and slippery paths and replace them with gentle ramps and all-weather surfaces? Are the doors into the garden and greenhouse wide enough? Consider narrowing borders so that you can reach them easily from the path. Raise as many of the beds as possible if you cannot bend, by getting retaining walls

Gardening from a wheelchair is made easier with long-handled handtools and safer if paths are wide and level.

built. Replace glass in greenhouses and frames with perspex for safety. Look at the type of tools available to help you. Nowadays it is possible to buy long-handled tools to use from a sitting or standing position. Always choose lightweight tools with aluminium, plastic or carbon-fibre handles. There are many tools with enlarged easy-grip handles and some can be adapted with strapping to use with one arm if necessary. If you are still able to dig but find it tiring (don't we all!), then use one of the long-handled spades or 'powered spades'; these throw off the earth by means of a hand-operated spring so that you do not have to bend.

Options for retirement

Consider whether your garden is too large to manage properly without overwork or worry. If it is, perhaps you can sell or let part of it, or have it converted from labour-intensive perennials to shrubs that are easier to manage. You might consider doing without a lawn and having the area paved so that your gardening can be done in raised beds and containers. Hedges require a lot of work and can be replaced by aesthetically pleasing fencing or trellis. Plan your garden for work little and often.

If you need regular access to a particular spot, consider installing handrails or grips to help you. Also, you should never forget the importance of easy watering. If you can use a hose then have a wall-mounted hosereel; if you are in a water-restricted area install standpipes you can easily reach with lightweight watering cans. If you enjoy fruit, grow cordon or espalier trained plants that you can pick without ladders or too much stretching or straining.

With some thought an existing garden can be adapted to your needs with relatively little expense. Practical tips and handy hints are available from some of the horticultural organizations. Addresses are given on page 157.

THE END OF THE DAY

○

'In puffs of balm the night-air blows
The perfume which the day fore-goes
And on the pure horizon far,
See, pulsing with the first-born star,
The liquid sky above the hill!
The evening comes, the fields are still.'
MATTHEW ARNOLD (1822–88)

Gardens have a particularly calming quality at the end of the day as the plants recover from heat and revive in the cool of the evening. This can often match our own moods as we recover from the stress and activity of the day, allowing the garden to refresh us spiritually.

Providing lighting in your garden can add a magical quality to this precious time of day. It can also enable you to see the activities of nocturnal animals and the roosting of birds, all of which link you with the natural world and its processes.

Sometimes you can almost see plants recover. From a slightly wilted appearance they succeed in drawing up water at a greater rate than they are losing it from their leaves. On the other hand, some plants 'go to sleep' by drooping their leaves in rest; this is a common phenomenon in shrubs belonging to the pea family.

Rest and regeneration

Rest is essential to the process of healing, both spiritually and physically. If we are deprived of sleep we suffer psychologically, and there is some evidence that we need a chance to dream, to review the past day and its conflicts and difficulties. There are many plants that can help us do just that, by enjoying their benefits in the form of herbal teas (see page 53) or using them to make a sweet-smelling pillow.

Each culture has its own image of eveningtide. The sounds and scents of a garden at the end of the day can be as evocative for an Arab in a garden in Marrakesh as for Matthew Arnold eulogizing the English evening and its promise of rest.

HOW TO MAKE A HERB PILLOW

Choose a pillowcase or cushion cover to suit the décor of your bedroom. Fill it with dried hop flowers, best obtained in the late autumn. Add a generous sprinkling of lavender flowers to the mixture and zip up the pillow. Place the pillow under your head to help you to sleep. The hop perfume induces sleep and the lavender is a relaxant. Refresh the mixture every few months by adding a few drops of essential oil of lavender to the mixture. Happy dreams!

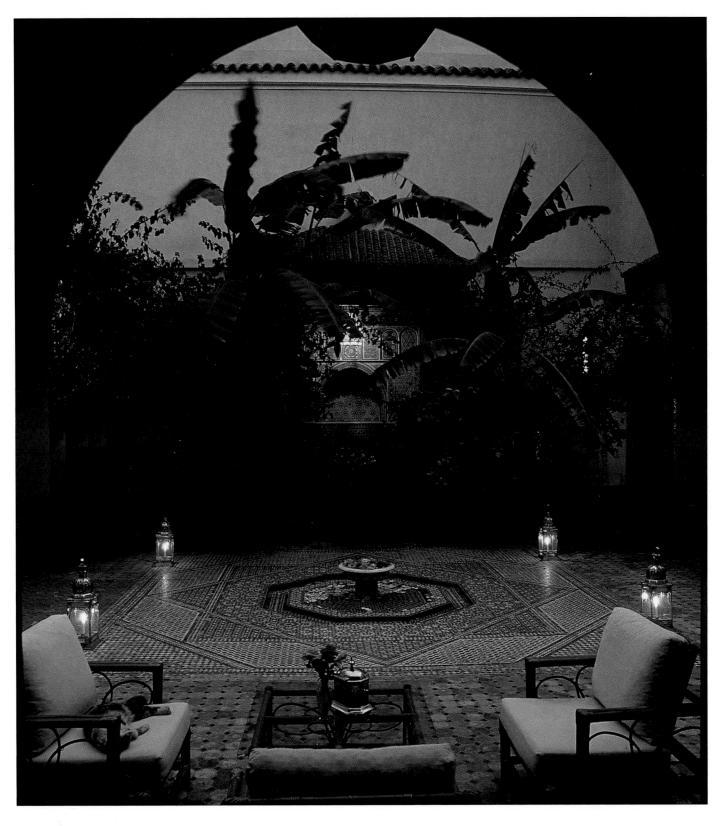

FURTHER READING

All publications are British unless otherwise noted.

CHAPTER ONE
The Healing Arts

Bensky and Gamble *Chinese Herbal Materia Medica* (Eastland Press, US, 1986).

Castro, M. *The Complete Homeopathy Handbook* (Macmillan, 1990).

Chishti, H. *The Traditional Healer* (Thorsons, 1988).

Cribb, A. B. and J. W. *Wild Medicine in Australia* (Angus and Robertson, Aust. 1992).

Nicholas Culpeper *Culpeper's Complete Herbal* (1653) (reprint Omega, 1985).

Grieve, M. *A Modern Herbal* (Penguin, 1978).

Griggs, B. *Green pharmacy: a history of herbal medicine* (Jill Norman and Hobhouse, 1981).

Hamilton, G. *Successful Organic Gardening* (Dorling Kindersley, 1987).

Heyn, B. *Ayurvedic Medicine* (Thorsons, 1987).

Hollman, A. Dr *Plants in Medicine* (Chelsea Physic Garden, 1991).

Kaptchuk, T. and Croucher, M. *The Healing Arts* (BBC Books, 1986).

Lovelock, James *Gaia: A New Look at Life on Earth* (OUP, 1979) and *The Ages of Gaia: a Biography of Our Living Planet* (OUP, 1988).

Stockwell, C. *Nature's Pharmacy* (Century, 1988).

CHAPTER TWO
The Body Physical

Baker, Harry *The Fruit Garden Displayed* (Royal Horticultural Society, 1991).

Boxer, A. and Back, P. *The Herb Book* (Octopus Books, 1980).

Buczacki, S. and Harris, K. *The Collins Guide to Pests, Diseases and Disorders of Garden Plants* (Collins, 1981).

Cowmeadow, O. *Introduction to Macrobiotics* (Thorsons, 1987).

Cartwright, Lorna *A Common Sense Guide to Medicinal Plants* (Angus and Robertson, Aust. 1985).

Deans, Esther *Esther Deans' Gardening Book* (Angus and Robertson, Aust. 1987).

Evans, M. *A Guide to Herbal Remedies* (C. W. Daniel, 1990) and *Herbal Plants* (Studio Editions, 1991).

Hayfield, Robin *Homeopathy for Common Ailments* (Angus and Robertson, Aust. 1992).

Larkom, Joy *The Salad Garden* (Windward, 1984), *The Vegetable Garden Displayed* (Royal Horticultural Society, 1992) and *Oriental Vegetables* (John Murray, 1991).

Lockie, A. Dr *The Family Guide to Homeopathy* (Elm Tree Books, 1989).

Leung, A. Y. *Encyclopedia of common natural ingredients used in food, drugs and cosmetics* (John Wiley, Chichester and New York, 1980).

Masefield, G. B., Wallis, M., Harrison, S. G. and Nicholson, B. E. *The Oxford Book of Food Plants* (Oxford University Press, 1979).

McIntyre, Anne *Herbs for Common Ailments* (Angus and Robertson, Aust. 1992).

Mitton, F. and Mitton, V. *Mitton's practical modern herbal* (Foulsham, 1982).

Polunin, M. and Robbins, C. *The Natural Pharmacy* (Dorling Kindersley, 1992).

Richardson, R. *The Little Garlic Book* (Piatkus, 1982).

Stevens, David *Making a Garden* (World Works, 1984).

Swanson, Faith *Herb Garden Design* (Hanover, NH, University Press of New England, 1984).

Wren, R. C. *Potter's New Cyclopaedia of Botanical Drugs and Preparations* (Daniel, 1988).

CHAPTER THREE
The Senses Awakened

Allison, J. *Water in the Garden* (Salamander Books, 1991).

Davis, P. *Aromatherapy, an A–Z* (C. W. Daniel, 1988).

Fleet, K. *Gardening without Sight* (RNIB, 1989).

Genders, R. *Scented Flora of the World, an Encyclopaedia* (Mayflower, Granada Publishing, 1978).

Hemphill, Rosemary *Cooking with Herbs and Spices* (Angus and Robertson, Aust. 1977), *Fragrance and Flavour* (Angus and Robertson, Aust. 1984), *Herbs for all Seasons* (Angus and Robertson, Aust. 1992).

Hobhouse, Penelope *Colour in Your Garden* (Collins, 1985; Boston, Little Brown, 1985).

Houdret, J. *Pomanders, Posies and Pot-pourri* (Shire, 1988).

Jekyll, Gertrude *Colour in the Flower Garden* (Country Life, 1908).

Lacey, Stephen *Scent in Your Garden* (Angus and Robertson, Aust. 1991).

Loewenfeld, C. and Back, P. *Herbs for health and cookery* (Pan Books, 1965).

Lloyd, Christopher *Foliage Plants* (Collins, 1973; Random House 1985).

Page, M. and Stearn, W. T. *Culinary herbs* (Wisley handbook 16, The Royal Horticultural Society, 1979).

Price, Shirley *Practical Aromatherapy* (Thorsons, 1987), *Aromatherapy for Common Ailments* (Angus and Robertson, Aust. 1992).

Wright, M. *The Complete Handbook of Garden Plants* (Michael Joseph, 1984).

Wrigley, John W. and Fagg, Murray *Aromatic Plants* from *The Australian Native Plant Library* (Angus and Robertson, Aust. 1990).

CHAPTER FOUR
A Spiritual Haven

Baines, C. *How to make a wildlife garden* (Elm Tree Books, 1985).

Banks, Elizabeth *Creating Period Gardens* (Phaidon, 1991).

Bazin, Germain *Paradeisos, The Art of the Garden* (Cassell, 1990).

Fisher, A. and Gerster, G. *The Art of the Maze* (Weidenfeld and Nicholson, 1990).

Hadfield, Miles *Topiary and Ornamental Hedges* (A. and C. Black, 1971).

Hagedorn, R. *Therapeutic Horticulture* (Winslow Press, 1987).

Hunt, Peter *The Book of Garden Ornaments* (Dent, 1974).

Jellicoe, G. A. and S. *The Landscape of Man* (Thames and Hudson, 1975).

Jellicoe, Goode and Lancaster *The Oxford Companion to Gardens* (Oxford University Press, 1991).

de Noailles, Vicomte and Lancaster, R. *Mediterranean Plants and Gardens* (Floraprint, 1990).

Please, P. (ed.) *Able to Garden: A Practical Guide for Disabled and Elderly Gardeners* (Batsford, 1990).

USEFUL ADDRESSES

American Horticultural Therapy Association, 9220 Wightman Road, Suite 300, Gaithersburgh, Maryland 20879, USA.

Australian Federation of Homeopaths Inc., PO Box 372, Balwyn, Vic. 3103.

Australian Herb Society, PO Box 110, Mapleton, Qld 4560.

Australian Institute of Homeopathy, 21 Bulah Close, Berowra Heights, NSW 2082.

The Dr Edward Bach Centre (Bach Flower Remedies), Mount Vernon, Sotwell, Wallingford, Oxon OX10 0PZ.

Brisbane Growers Group Inc., PO Box 236, Intwyche, Qld 4030.

British Herbal Medicine Association, Lane House, Cowling, Keighley, W. Yorks BD22 0LX.

Chelsea Physic Garden, 66 Royal Hospital Road, London SW3 4HS.

Henry Doubleday Research Association (information on organic gardening),

Ryton Gardens, Ryton-on-Dunsmore, Coventry CV8 3LG.

Henry Doubleday Research Association of Australia Inc., 816 Comleroy Road, Kurrajong, NSW 2758 (organic gardening, biodynamics, permaculture).

Ecological Society of Australia, PO Box 1564, Canberra, ACT 2601.

Gardening for Disabled Trust, Church Cottage, Headcorn, Kent TN27 9NP.

The Herb Society, 34 Boscobel Place, London SW1W 9PE.

Kushi Institute (Macrobiotic classes), 188 Old Street, London EC1V 9BP.

Macrobiotics International, 17 Station Street, Brookline, MA 02147, USA.

National Herbalists Association of Australia, PO Box 65, Kingsgrove, NSW 2208.

National Institute of Medical Herbalists, 148, Forest Road, Tunbridge Wells, Kent TN2 5EY.

Permaculture International, PO Box 7185, Lismore Heights, NSW 2480.

Permaculture Association of Western Australia, PO Box 148, Inglewood, WA 6052.

Royal Blind Society, 4 Mitchell Road, Enfield, NSW 2136.

Royal National Institute for the Blind, 224 Portland Street, London W1N 6AA.

Royal Society for the Protection of Birds (RSPB), The Lodge, Sandy, Bedfordshire SG19 2DL.

Ryde College of Technical and Further Education – Telopea Centre, 250 Blaxland Road, Ryde, NSW 2112.

Soil Association (for information on organic gardening), 86 Colston Street, Bristol BS1 5BB.

Trust for Urban Ecology (TRUE), Stave Hill Ecological Park, Timberpond Road, London SE16 1AG.

LIST OF SUPPLIERS

Herbs – seeds and plants

BRITAIN

Norfolk Lavender Ltd, Caley Mill, Heacham, King's Lynn, Norfolk. *Plants.*

Old Rectory Herb Garden, Ightham, Nr Sevenoak, Kent. *Plants only.*

Suffolk Herbs, Monk's Farm, Pantlings Lane, Kelvedon, Essex CO5 9PG. *Organically grown herbs and seeds.*

The Herb Garden, Thunderbridge, Nr Huddersfield, Yorks. *Plants.*

Tresare Herb Farm, Taman Bay, Looe, Cornwall. *SAE with enquiries.*

USA (seeds only)

Comstock, Ferre and Co., 263 Main Street, Wethersfield, Conn 06109.

Rocky Hollow Herb Farm Inc., R.D.2, Box 215, Lake Wallkill Road, Sussex, NJ 07461.

CANADA (seeds only)

Otto Richter and Sons Ltd, Locust Hill, Ontario, Canada LO4 1J0.

AUSTRALIA

Broersen Seeds and Bulbs Pty Ltd, Monbulk-Silvan Road, Silvan, Vic. 3795. *Seeds.*

Eden Seeds, Mail Service 316, Gympie, Qld 4570. *Organic seeds.*

Meadow Herbs, Sims Road, Mt Barker, SA 5251.

Rose-World Nursery Pty Ltd, Redland Bay Road, Victoria Point, Qld 4163. *Plants.*

Swanes Nursery, 490 Galston Road, Dural, NSW 2158.

NEW ZEALAND

Arthur Yates and Co. Ltd, 270 Neilson Street, Onehunga, Auckland. *Seeds.*

Kings Herb Nursery, 17a Methuen Road, Avondale, Auckland. *Plants and seeds.*

Organic control of pests

English Woodland Ltd, Burrow Nursery, Cross in Hand, Heathfield, E. Sussex TN21 0UG.

Koppert (UK) Ltd, 1 Wadhurst Business Park, Faircrouch Lane, Wadhurst, E. Sussex TN5 6PT.

Water gardening

Stapeley Water Gardens Ltd, Stapeley, Nantwich, Cheshire CW5 7LH.

Maydencroft Aquatic Nurseries, Maydencroft Lane, Gosmore, Hitchin, Herts.

Aromatherapy oils and suppliers

Culpeper Ltd, 21 Bruton Street, London W1X 7DA.

Period garden furniture and trompe l'oeil

Andrew Crace Designs, 51 Bourne Lane, Much Hadham, Herts. SG10 6ER.

Terracotta pots

Pots and Pithoi (importer), Grange Farm, Turners Hill Road, Crawley Down, West Sussex.

Whichford Potteries, Whichford, Shipston-on-Stour, Warwickshire CV36 5PG.

Unusual and tender plants

Chiltern Seeds, Bortree Stile, Ulverston, Cumbria LA12 7PB.

Gould Farm Nurseries, Frittenden, Cranbrook, Kent TN17 2DT.

Hopley's Plants Ltd, High Street, Much Hadham, Herts. SG10 6BU.

Refer also to nurseries listed in:
Tony Lord (ed.) *The Plant Finder* published yearly by Headmain Ltd.

Wildflowers – seeds and plants

John Chambers, 15 Westleigh Road, Barton Seagrave, Kettering, Northamptonshire NN15 5AJ.

Landlife Wild Flowers Ltd, The Old Police Station, Lark Lane, Liverpool L17 8UU.

INDEX

Page numbers in *italics* indicate captions to illustrations

A

Acer (Maple) 114
Achillea 58, 89, 115
acne 61
acupuncture 13
Africa 15
AIDS 27
allantoin 64
allicin 48
allopathic medicine 22
allyl isothiocyanate 81
Althaea (Marsh Mallow) 58
American Indians 15
anatomy 11, 12
Angelica 72
Anise 72
antimony 12
Antirrhinum 115
anxiety 32
Apothecaries' Garden of
    Simples 18-19
appetite, stimulating 59
Apples 43, *43*
Apricots 43
aquatic plants, marginal 135
Aristotle 10, 12
aromatherapy 62, 70, 104,
    110-11
arrow poison 24
arsenic 22
Artemisia 13, *13*, *31*, 58
artemisinin 58
arterial disorders 32, 34
arthritis 59
Artichokes 47
Arum 102
Asparagus *39*, 45
aspirin 59
astrology 12, 28
Aubergine 47
Australia 14, 15
Avicenna 11, 110
Ayurveda 14-15, 34
Aztecs 15

B

Bach Flower Remedies 66-7
Bamboo *96*
barks, textured 114
Basil 70, 72, 76
Bay (*Laurus*) 73, *78*, 122, 131
bereavement 27
Bergamot 52, 53, 73
Betula (Birch) 114, *115*
birds, attracting 116
Blackberries 42, 43
bleeding, staunching 58

blind and partially sighted,
    garden for 116-17, *116*
blood circulation 65
blood pressure, high 64
blood-letting 12, 22
blue schemes 85, 88-91
Blueberries 42
Borage 73
botanic gardens 12, 16
Box (*Buxus*) *92*, 122, 128, 131,
    131
brassicas, unusual 45-7
Bridgeman, Charles 132
bronchial problems 60, 81
Brown, 'Capability' 132
bruises 64
Brunfels, Otto 20
Buddhism 124
Buddleja 122
butterflies, attracting 122,
    144, 145

C

Cabbage, red *38*, *39*
Calendula (Marigold) *31*, 32
Camomile (*Chamaemelum*) 32,
    52, 53
Campanula 91
Cananga 110
cancer 27, 32, 59, 61
Cape gooseberry 45
Caraway 73
carbenoxalone 60
cardiology 59
Cassia senna 12
castanospermine 27
castor oil 10
Castor Oil Plant (*Ricinus*) 58,
    62, *62*
Catharanthus 18, 32, 65-6
Cauliflower 40
Cayenne Pepper 65
Celeriac 45
Centaurea 115
Centaurium (Centaury) 58
Chelsea Physic Garden *16*,
    17, 18-19, *19*, 97, 109,
    150
chemicals, from plants 20
Cherries 43
Chervil 73, 78
chest infections 58
chillblains 81
Chilli Pepper 65
chills 81
China 13, 16
Chinese gooseberry 44

Chinese greens 47
Chives 73
Christianity 12, 124
Cinchona 18
Cistus 114
Citrus 52
Clematis 66, *94*
cocaine 15
codeine 32, 61, 63
colchicine 59
colour wheel 83
colours 82-91
    complementary 88-91
    groupings 86-7
    mood and 84-5
    use 83
Comfrey 64
companion planting 36, 39
compost, garden 37, 38
compost, potting 37
conservation 24
constipation 62
containers *92*, 150
contraceptives 24, 63
Coral Tree (*Erythrina*) 150
Coriander 40, 73, 77
cottage gardens *127*, 132
coughs 58, 61
Cowslip (*Primula*) 61
Culpeper, Nicholas 12, 20,
    21, 52, 58, 59, 64
Cumin 73-4
Curare 15, 24, *24*
Currants *32*, 42, 43

D

Dahlia 115
derris 39
diabetics 47
diarrhoea 62
diet, healthy 34-5
digestion 32, 58, 59
digging 37
Digitalis (Foxglove) 59, *63*
digitoxin 59
digoxin 59, 63
Dill 74
Dioscorea 24
Dioscorides 11, 12, 16, *21*
disabled, gardening for 153,
    153
diseases of crops 39
Doctrine of Signatures 18,
    60, 64, 65, 66
drugs, related to plants 24,
    63
dysentery 62, 66

E

ecology 28
eczema 32, 50, 61
Egypt 10, 16
Elder (*Sambucus*) 58, 64
elderly, gardening for 153
Elecampane (*Inula*) 61
Eucalyptus 70
Evening Primrose 32, *50*, 61
expectorants 70

F

facial treatments 119
fats, in food 34
Fennel *32*, 74, 77, 78
fever 15, 32, 64
Feverfew (*Tanacetum*) *32*, 64
fibre, in food 34
Fig (*Ficus*) 44
flora, saving 24
folk medicine 14-15
foot massage 119
Fortune, Robert 18
fountains 96, *99*, *100*, 116,
    116
fractures 64
Frankincense 110
French Marigolds *36*
Friar's Balsam 104
fruit 42-5
    tropical, from pips 46
Fuchs, Leonard 20
fumigation 12, 112

G

Gages 43
Gaia 28
Galen 11
gamma-linolenic acid 61
gardens
    design 127-9
    dry 149
    enclosed 124, *124*
    formal 127-9, *128*
    informal 127
    romantic 127, 134-3
    secret 123, *124*
Garlic (*Allium*) 32, 48-9, *49*
Gelsemium 66
genetic research 59
Gentiana 59
geophysiology 28
Gerard, John 20, *21*, 64,
    112
germicides 104
Ginger (*Zingiber*) 20, 66

Giverny, France *136*
glaucoma 22, 24
Glendurgan, Cornwall *139*
Gooseberries 42, 43
gout 32, 58, 59
Grape Vine *122*
Greeks 11, 16
green schemes 84, *85*
grey foliage *82*
Gunnera 92

H
Hahnemann, Dr Samuel 22
Hawthorn (*Crataegus*) 58, 59
headaches 32, 59, 61, 70
healing, ancient art 10-11
hearing, features pleasing to
    96-101, 116
heart 24, 59, 65
hedgehogs 145
hedges 92, 129, 144-5
Hemerocallis 82
herb garden *31*, 54-6, 92
herb pillow 154
herb wheel 55, *55*
herbal teas 52-3
herbalism 20, 27
herbals 20, *21*
herbs 78, *78*, 112
    for kitchen 72-7
    medicinal 20, 50-1
    for scenting air 112-13
heroin 61
Hippocrates 12, 22
Hodgkin's disease 18
holistic medicine 20, 22, 27
homoeopathy 22-3, 27
Honesty (*Lunaria*) 115
Honeysuckle (*Lonicera*) 70
Hop (*Humulus*) 53, 58, 60
hormonal imbalance 65
Horsetail 53
'Hortus Clusianus' 17, *17*
humours 10-11, *11*, 12-13,
    14-15
Hutton, James 28
hyoscine 15, 60
hyperactivity 34

I
Ice Plants 114
immune deficiency diseases
    27
Impatiens 115
Incas 15
India 14
indigestion 32, 60
infection 32
inflammation 32, 58
insects, attracting 96-7, 145
Islam 124

J
Japan 13
Japanese gardens *99*, *121*,
    148-9, *148*
Jasminum 70, *107*
Jekyll, Gertrude 56, 82, 88,
    127, 132
Jellicoe, Sir Geoffrey 147
Jesuits' Bark 18
Juniperus 70

K
Kampo 13
kidney 59, 61, 65
Kiwi fruit 44
knot gardens 92, 130
Kohlrabi 47

L
labdanum 114
lactic acid 118
Ladew Topiary Garden *130*
lakes 134
landscapes 92, 132
Lavandula (Lavender) *31*, 70,
    109, *109*
laxatives, earliest 10
leaves *85*, 114
Lemon Balm (*Melissa*) 52, 53
Lemon Verbena (*Aloysia*) *32*,
    53, 74
Leonardo da Vinci 12, 88
Lettuce 40, *41*
leukemia 18, 32, 66
Levens Hall, Cumbria *131*
lighting 141, 154
Lilium 69, *82*, *94*, *104*, *122*
Lime blossom 53
Liquorice (*Glycyrrhiza*) 60
liver 58
Loganberries 42, 43
loofah (*Luffa*) 118-19
Loquat 44
Lovage 74
Lovelock, James 28
lungs 61
Lysimachia (Creeping Jenny)
    91

M
macrobiotics 35
Magnolia 104
malaria 18, 58
Male Fern (*Dryopteris*) 59, *59*
Mandrake 60, *60*, 61
marginal plants 135
Marjoram 74
massage 118-19
Mayans 15
mazes 138-9, *138*, *139*
Meadow Saffron (*Colchicum*)
    32, *58*, 59

Meadowsweet (*Filipendula*) 59
medicinal plants *32*, 58-66
medicine, beginnings 10
Mediterranean garden 150-1
Medlar 44
Melilotus (Melilot) 58, 61
menopause 65
mercury 12
Mesopotamia 10
methyl salicylate 65
migraine 32, 64, 66
Miller, Philip 18, 109
Mint 52, 53, 75, *119*
monasteries 16
Monet, Claude, garden *136*
mood, effect of colour on
    84-5
morning sickness 66
morphine 32, 61
motion sickness 20, 63, 66
moxa 13
moxibustion 13
Mulberry 44-5, *44*
mulching 37
Muscari 107
muscle relaxants 24
Mustard 80-1
Myosotis 88
Myrrh 110

N
Narcissus 107
Nasturtium 75
Nectarines 43
nervous exhaustion 64
neuralgia 66, 81
New Zealand 14, 15, 132
Nicotiana (Tobacco Plant) *70*,
    102, *104*, 106

O
oils
    essential 110-11, 112
    for massage 118-19
Okra 45
Onions *40*
Opium Poppy (*Papaver*) *32*,
    58, 61, *61*
orange schemes *85*, 86-7
Oregano 74
organic gardening 37-8
Orris 60, 112
Oswego Tea 52
Oxford Physic Garden 17

P
painkillers 60
papain 65
Paracelsus 12, 16
paralysis 22
Parkinson, John 58
Parsley 75

paths 128-9
Pawpaw (Papaya) 65
Peaches 43
Pears 43
Pelargonium 70, *114*, 116
perfumery 62, 112
Persimmon 44
pests in garden 39
physic gardens 16-17
physiology 11
physostigmine 24
pilocarpine 24, 63
pink schemes *82*, 84
pituitary gland 65
plague 12, 112
Plums 43
Podophyllum 61
pollution 27
pomanders 112
Pomegranate 45, *45*
pools 134-6, 144
pot-pourri 112-13
potager 129, *129*
Potatoes 40-1
Potentilla 89
poultices 64, 81
pregnancy 64
premenstrual tension 32, 61,
    65
Primula 61
Privet 131
Prunus 114
psychoneuroimmunology 27
psychosomatic illness 27
purgatives 64
purple foliage 86
Purslane 75
Pyracantha 102
pyrethrum 39

Q
quaiacum 12
Quassia 66
Quercus 114
Quince 44
quinine 12, 15, 18

R
rainforests 24
Raspberries 42, 43
recipes 49, 76-7, 78, 81
red schemes 84, 86-7
religious symbols *122*
remedies for minor ills 51
Renaissance 12
Repton, Humphry 132
Rheum 62
rheumatic complaints 15, 81
Robinson, William 127
Romans 11
Rosa (Rose) 58, 62, *62*, 70,
    112, *119*, *132*

old *102*, 132-3
rose hips 53, 62
Rosemary 70, 75, 78, 112
Rosemary oil 50
Rue 112
runner beans *36*
ruptures 64

S

Sackville-West, Vita 94
Sage 53, 75, 78
salicylic acid 59
Salix 96
Salsify 47
Salvia 114, *see also* Sage
Santolina 92
Savory (*Satureja*) 75
scent 102-13, 116-17
    classification 105
    in conservatory 107
Scorzonera 47
sculpture 140-2, *140, 141,*
    143
scurvy 32
Seakale 47, *47*
sedatives 64
Sedum 144
seedheads 114-15
self-expression 147
Senna 10, 12, 66
senses, stimulating 69-119
shape, plants for 92-3
Sharon fruit 44
shell gardens 147

shingle garden 147
sight, plants to please 82-91
Sisal 119
skin problems 60, 61
Skullcap (*Scutellaria*) 64
sleep, inducing 60, 154
Sloane, Sir Hans 18, *18*
Snowdrops 107
snuff 60, 81, 112
Society of Apothecaries
    18-19
Sorbus (Rowan) *122*
sounds, healing 96-101
spiritual haven 121-54
Sri Lanka 14-15
steroids 24, 63
stomach 65
Strawberries 42, 43
Strelitzia (Bird of Paradise) 150
stress 27
Strophanthus 24, *24*
structure, plants for 92-3
Strychnos 22
Styrax 104
sundial *9*
Sweet Cicely 75
Sweet Peppers 47
symptoms, attitudes to 22
syphilis 12

T

Tagetes 39
Tamarillo 44
Tarragon 75, 78

taste, plants for 72-81, 116
Tayberries 42, 43
Tea 18, 65
teas, herbal 52-3
textures, in plants 114-15
Theophrastus 11, *21*
theophylline 65
therapy of gardening 153
throat, sore 62
thrombosis 61
Thyme 52, 53, 75, 78, *106,*
    112
tobacco 12, 15, 81
toothache 81
topiary 130-1, *130,* 147
touch, planting for 114-19
trompe-l'oeil 142, *142*
Tropaeolum 75, 82
tuberculosis 61
Tuberose (*Polianthes*) 107
tubocurarine *24*
Tulip 88

U

ulcers 60, 64
urine, diagnosis from 12

V

Valerian *32*, 53, 64
vegetables 40-1, 45-7
vegetarianism 34-5
Veratrum 64
Verbascum 31, 53
Verbena (Vervain) 64-5

vermifuge 59
Villandry 129, *129*
Vinca 18
Viola 65, *65*
Virgin Mary 124
Vitex 58, 65

W

Wardian cases 18
water in garden 96, 99-101,
    134-7
waterfalls 96, 100, *100*
Water lilies 114
weeds 37-9
white schemes 94-5
wildlife garden 144-5, *145*
Wisley, RHS gardens 31
Witch Hazel (*Hamamelis*) 58,
    60
woodland 145
Woodruff (*Galium*) 53
worms 32, 59
wounds 32

Y

yellow schemes 84-5, 88-91
Yew (*Taxus*) 122, 131, *131*
yin and yang 35
Ylang-ylang *110*

Z

Zen Buddhist garden 148,
    149

○

AUTHOR ACKNOWLEDGEMENTS

Many thanks are due to Penny Hammond for considerable feedback and assistance; Dr Arthur Hollman for advice and technical information on double-blind tested drugs; Susyn Andrews for taxonomic assistance on lavenders; the Wellcome Galleries of the History of Medicine; Roy Genders for his work towards classification of plant perfumes; J. and J. Colman of Norwich, England, for information on the history of mustard; Penelope Hobhouse for her pioneering work on the history of colour; and Celia Toler, Maureen O'Grady and Alistair Aitken for typing.

The plan of the Chelsea Physic Garden on page 19 is reprinted by kind permission of The Royal Society.

The table on page 63 owes much to the work of Dr Arthur Hollman of the Royal College of Physicians of London and Adviser to the Chelsea Physic Garden.

The recipe for Welsh Rarebit on page 81 is kindly supplied by Messrs. J and J. Colman of Norwich, England.

The table on page 105 is based on Roy Genders' *Scented Flora of the World: An Encyclopaedia* (1978).

The recipe for pot-pourri on page 113 is reprinted from *The Book of the Rose* by Michael Gibson (Macdonald, 1980).

EDDISON·SADD

Photographs

T = TOP B = BELOW C = CENTRE
L = LEFT R = RIGHT
Sue Atkinson 26, 48, 74T, 82, 88, 91, 115; Trygve Boistad/Panos Pictures 35; Linda Burgess/The Garden Picture Library 49; Neil Campbell-Sharp/Trip 40, 52, 54. 63T, 108, 119R, 144; The Chelsea Physic Garden 12, 16, 18, 19L and R, 21, 22, 45, 109; Geoff Dawn/The Garden Picture Library 145; Liz Eddison 2, 6, 8-9, 47, 60, 62L, 63B, 73L & R, 75, 76, 79, 98, 99, 101, 104L & C, 113, 114, 117; Mary Evans 10, 11, 13T, 28; John Glover 29, 30-31, 36, 39, 41, 58, 59, 62R, 68-69, 73C, 74B, 92L, 96R, 102-103, 107, 125, 126, 128, 134, 146; Jerry Harpur 34, 38, 42, 43, 56, 83, 85, 106, 129, 130, 142, 150, 152, 155; Marijke Heuff/The Garden Picture Library 96L; Neil Holmes/The Garden Picture Library 118; The Hutchison Library 13B, 14, 25; Andrew Lawson 44, 50T & B, 65, 72, 94, 100, 131, 132,

138; Frank Leather/Trip 148; Tania Midgley 55, 92R, 104R, 120-121, 135, 139, 141, 143; Sue Minter/The Chelsea Physic Garden 86, 140; Oxford Scientific Films 24; Jerry Pavia/The Garden Picture Library 57, 149; The Harry Smith Collection 66, 80, 81, 119L; Perdereau Thomas/The Garden Picture Library 136; May Woods/The Garden Picture Library 17

Project Editor Geraldine Christy
Art Director Elaine Partington
Designer Sarah Howerd
Illustrator Lynn Chadwick
Picture Researcher Liz Eddison
Indexer Dorothy Frame
Production Hazel Kirkman and Charles James